Ocular Surface Diseases
- Some Current Date on Tear Film Problem and Keratoconic Diagnosis

Edited by Dorota Kopacz

Published in London, United Kingdom

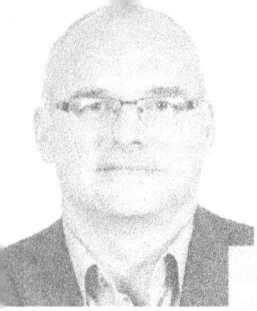
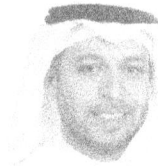
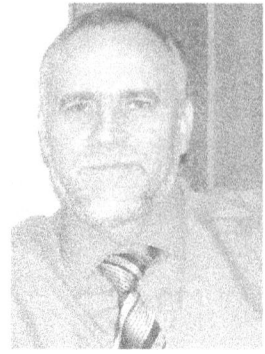
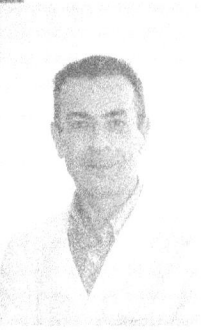
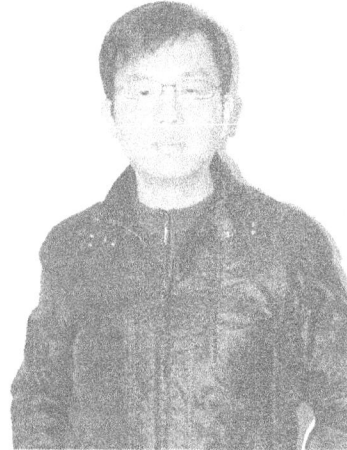
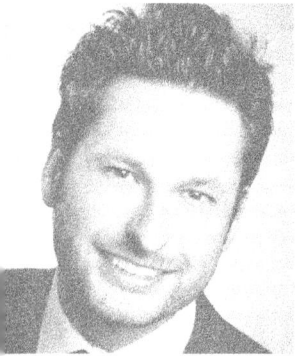
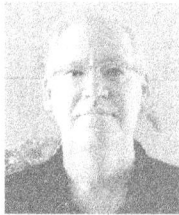

IntechOpen

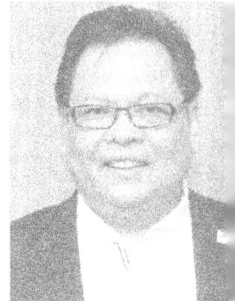
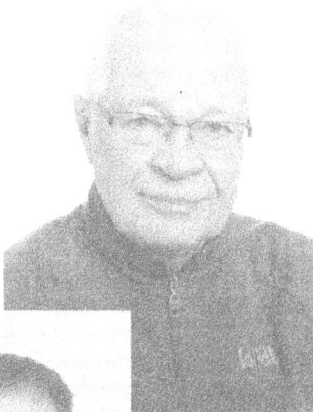
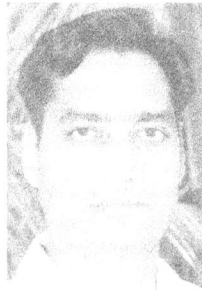
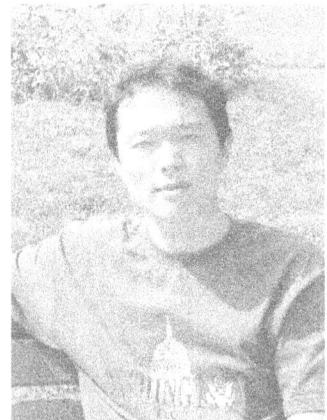
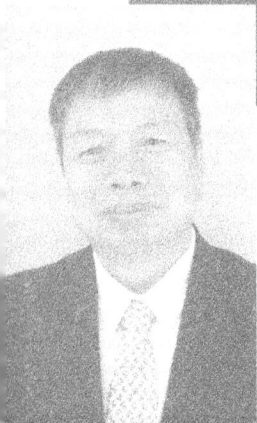
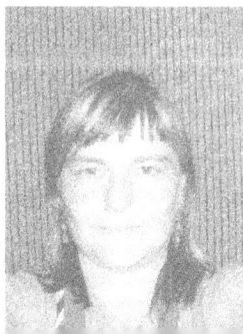

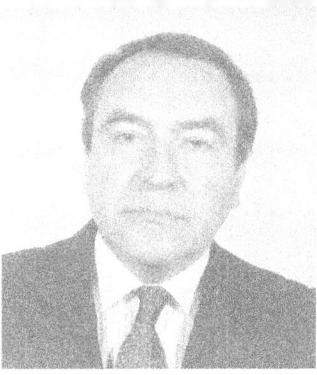

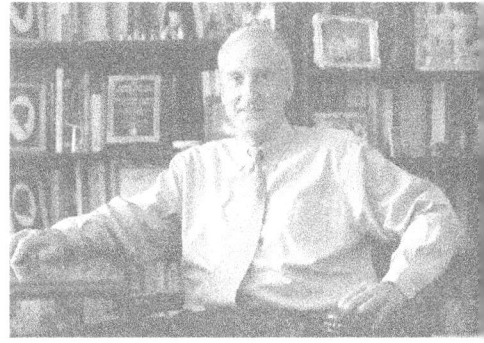

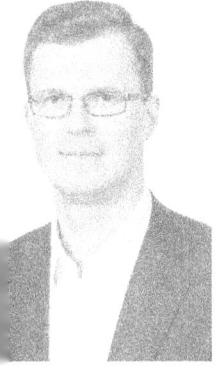

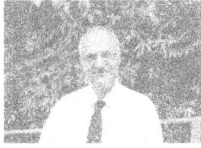

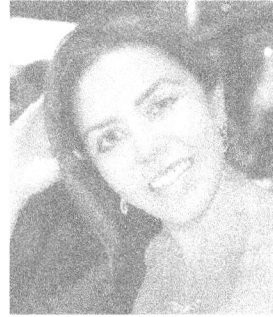

Supporting open minds since 2005

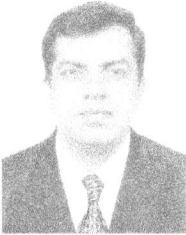

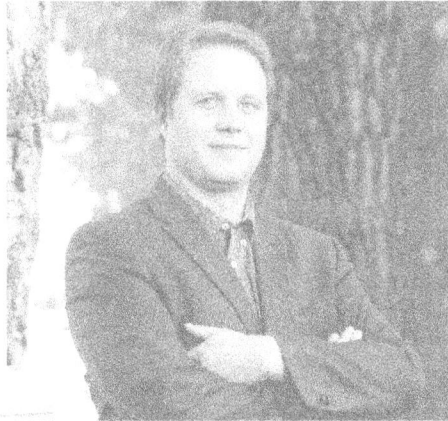

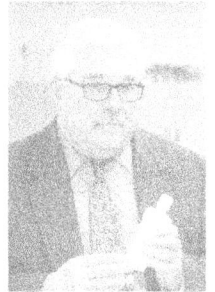

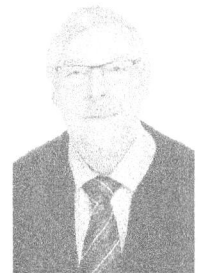

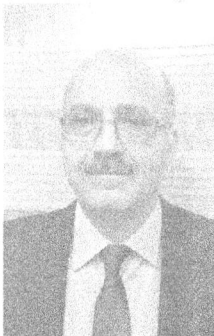

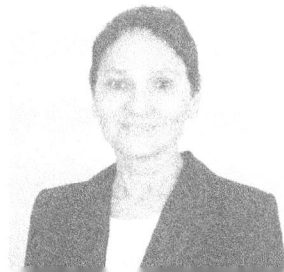

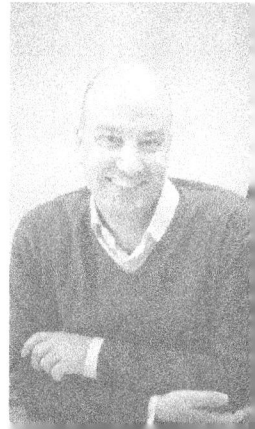

Ocular Surface Diseases - Some Current Date on Tear Film Problem and Keratoconic Diagnosis
http://dx.doi.org/10.5772/intechopen.77516
Edited by Dorota Kopacz

Contributors
Henry D. Perry, Maria Vincent, Jose Quintero, James Rynerson, Alejandro Aguilar, Alejandro Berra, Juan Wang, Calvin C.P. Pang, Yu Meng Wang, Dorota Kopacz

Notice
Statements and opinions expressed in the chapters are these of the individual contributors and not necessarily those of the editors or publisher. No responsibility is accepted for the accuracy of information contained in the published chapters. The publisher assumes no responsibility for any damage or injury to persons or property arising out of the use of any materials, instructions, methods or ideas contained in the book.

First published in London, United Kingdom, 2021 by IntechOpen
IntechOpen is the global imprint of INTECHOPEN LIMITED, registered in England and Wales, registration number: 11086078, 5 Princes Gate Court, London, SW7 2QJ, United Kingdom
Printed in Croatia

British Library Cataloguing-in-Publication Data
A catalogue record for this book is available from the British Library

Additional hard and PDF copies can be obtained from orders@intechopen.com

Ocular Surface Diseases - Some Current Date on Tear Film Problem and Keratoconic Diagnosis
Edited by Dorota Kopacz
p. cm.
Print ISBN 978-1-83880-959-1
Online ISBN 978-1-83880-960-7
eBook (PDF) ISBN 978-1-83880-961-4

We are IntechOpen,
the world's leading publisher of
Open Access books
Built by scientists, for scientists

5,100+
Open access books available

127,000+
International authors and editors

145M+
Downloads

156
Countries delivered to

Our authors are among the
Top 1%
most cited scientists

12.2%
Contributors from top 500 universities

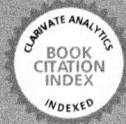

CLARIVATE ANALYTICS
BOOK
CITATION
INDEX
INDEXED

WEB OF SCIENCE™

Selection of our books indexed in the Book Citation Index
in Web of Science™ Core Collection (BKCI)

Interested in publishing with us?
Contact book.department@intechopen.com

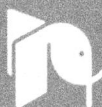

Meet the editor

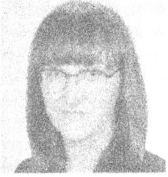

Dorota Kopacz MD, Ph.D., is professionally connected with the Department of Ophthalmology, Medical University of Warsaw, Poland, where she is a tutor for medical, dentistry, and rescue students; a tutor for doctors during specialization in general practice, diabetology, rheumatology, and ophthalmology; and a thesis supervisor for bachelor's degrees. She is also a consulting ophthalmologist at Infant Jesus Teaching Hospital, Warsaw, Poland. Protector for doctors during specialization in ophthalmology. Dr. Kopacz is a member of the Polish Society of Ophthalmology, European Society of Cataract and Refractive Surgery, and Cornea Society. Her clinical experience includes diagnostic procedures and non-invasive ophthalmological treatment (especially of the anterior eye segment and ocular surface), cataract surgery, secondary intraocular lens implantations, glaucoma, and ocular surface problems. She is author/coauthor of more than 160 publications, book chapters, congress papers, and posters. She is also a reviewer for local and international ophthalmological journals.

Contents

Preface

Many studies have been performed to describe and to understand the correlations between the structures of the eye, also known as the "ocular surface." This book focuses on the preocular tear film, a thin layer of tears covering the cornea of the eye. It presents research on tear film physiology, its changes in various disturbances and diseases, and the influence of those changes on the ocular surface. It also presents up-to-date information on keratoconus, a condition affecting both the preocular tear film and the ocular surface in which the cornea thins and bulges outward.

This book was made possible thanks to the collaboration of many researchers in the field of ophthalmology. I wish to thank them as well as the staff at IntechOpen for their invaluable contributions. I hope ophthalmologists, practitioners, and students will find this book interesting and useful for understanding the role of preocular tear film in ocular surface integrity and stability.

Dr. Dorota Kopacz
Medical University of Warsaw,
Warsaw, Poland

Department of Ophthalmology,
Infant Jesus Teaching Hospital,
Warsaw, Poland

Chapter 1

Tear Film – Physiology and Disturbances in Various Diseases and Disorders

Dorota Kopacz, Łucja Niezgoda, Ewa Fudalej,
Anna Nowak and Piotr Maciejewicz

Abstract

The tear film is a thin fluid layer covering the ocular surface. It is responsible for ocular surface comfort, mechanical, environmental and immune protection, epithelial health and it forms smooth refractive surface for vision. The traditional description of the tear film divides it into three layers: lipid, aqueous and mucin. The role of each layer depends on the composition of it. Tear production, evaporation, absorption and drainage concur to dynamic balance of the tear film and leads to its integrity and stability. Nonetheless, this stability can be disturb in tear film layers deficiencies, defective spreading of the tear film, in some general diseases and during application of some general and/or topical medications. Dry eye disease is the result of it. In this review not only physiology of the tear film is presented. Moreover, we would like to discuss the influence of various diseases and conditions on the tear film and contrarily, spotlight tear film disorders as a manifestation of those diseases.

Keywords: tear film, dry eye, mucins, lipid layer, aqueous layer, ocular surface

1. Introduction

The tear film is a thin fluid layer covering the ocular surface; it is the interface of the ocular surface with the environment. It is responsible for ocular surface comfort, mechanical, environmental and immune protection, epithelial (both corneal and conjunctival) health and it forms smooth, refracting surface for vision [1, 2]. Tear production (about 1,2 microliters per minute, total volume 6 microliters, 16% turnover per minute), evaporation, absorption and drainage are responsible for dynamic balance of the preocular tear film [1, 3–5]. Homeostatic balance leads to stability of the tear film, that makes possible to realize its functions as lubrication, nutrition and protection of ocular surface [3, 6]. Nonetheless, this stability can be disturb in tear film layers deficiencies, defective spreading of the tear film, in some general diseases and during application of some systemic and/or topical medications and dry eye disease evolves as a consequence of it. These review focused on physiology of the tear film, it's meaning for the ocular surface stability and analyzed influence of various diseases and conditions on it.

2. Tear film structure and function

The traditional description of the tear film is three-layered structure: super-ficial-oily, middle - aqueous and mucous layer at the base [1–3]. A more recently proposed model consists of two layers: superficial – lipids and mucin/aqueous glycocalyx gel with decreasing mucin concentration from epithelium to lipid layer [1, 3, 7, 8]. Some authors says, that the tear film is a single unit that acts like a fluid shell [9] (**Table 1** and **Figure 1**).

Tear film layer	Function
Lipid layer (meibum)	• Form the outer layer of the tear film. • Minimize the evaporation of water from the eye surface • Isolate ocular surface from the environment • Improve the stability of tear film • Provide smooth refracting surface • Limit contamination of ocular surface from particles(dust) and microorganisms • Prevent tear contamination by skin lipids • Limit aqueous layer surface tension • Counteract tears overflowing onto the skin
Aqueous phase	• Constitutes roughly 90% of the tear film volume • Lubricate the ocular surface • Wash away foreign bodies and contaminations • Nourish the avascular cornea (oxygen, proteins, inorganic salts) • Include proteins (lysozyme, lactoferrin, lipocain), immunoglobulins, defensins and glycoproteins responsible for anti-microbial activity • Include growth factors, vitamins and electrolytes necessary for ocular surface health and epithelial integrity • Realign corneal microirregularities (refractive properties)
Mucous layer	• Form a glycocalyx over the ocular epithelium that prevents pathogen adhesion • Bind water to hydrate and lubricate the ocular surface. • Reduce friction during blinking • Clear the surface of pathogens and debris • Contribute to tear stability • Take part in regulation of epithelial growth • Might be involved in cellular signaling

Table 1.
The function of tear film layers.

2.1 Lipids

The lipid layer is secreted by Meibomian glands, located within tarsal plates of upper and lower eyelids with some small contribution by Moll (modified apocrinic, sudoriferous) and Zeiss (modified subeceous) glands, located within superior and lower eyelids (connected with hair follicles) and possibly epithelial cells. The posterior, aqueous interface consists of polar lipids: ceramides, cerebrosides and phospholipids. The lipid-air interface is formed with nonpolar lipids: cholesterol esters, triglycerides and free fatty acids [1, 3, 7, 8, 10].

The main function of the lipid layer is to reduce evaporation of tears and improve the stability of them. Moreover, the lipid layer provides smooth refracting surface, limits contamination of ocular surface from particles (dust) and microor-ganisms, prevents tear contamination by skin lipids, limits aqueous layer surface tension and counteracts tears overflowing onto the skin. [1, 3, 7–14].

Regulation of lipid secretion supervenes through modulation of lipid synthesis or cell maturation. The Meibomian gland secretion is a subject of neuronal, hormonal

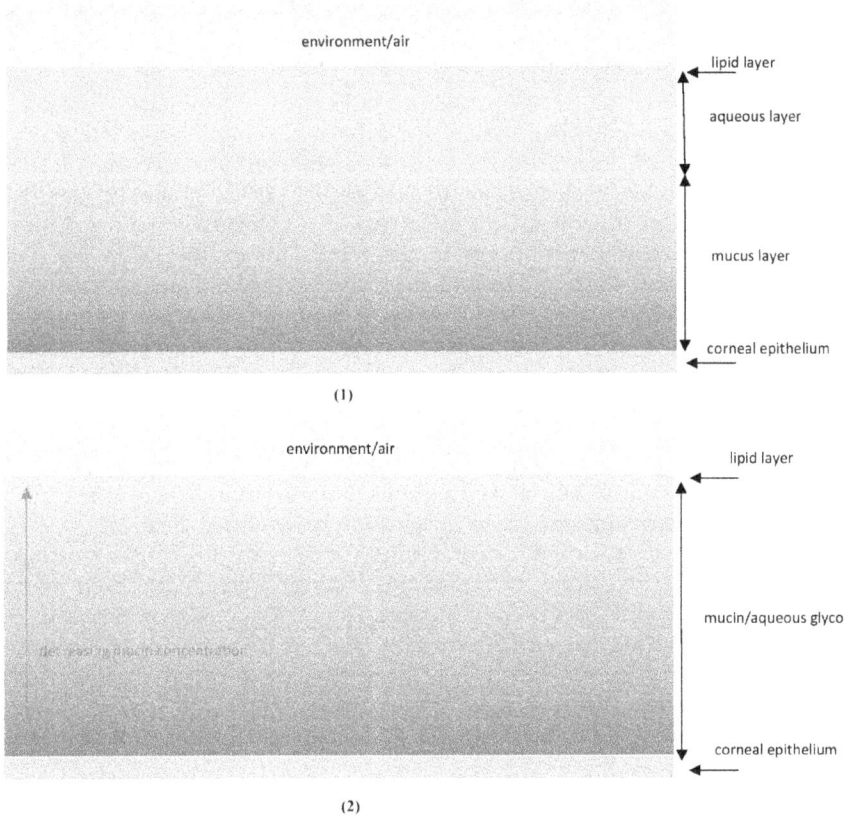

Figure 1.
Structure of the tear film: 1. Three layer conception. 2. Two layer conception.

and vascular influences. Androgen, estrogen and progesterone receptors have been identified in adult male and female rats, rabbits and humans. It is suggested that androgens stimulate and estrogens reduce Meibomian secretion [14–17]. Moreover, Meibomian gland function may be under direct neuronal (predominant parasympathetic, also sympathetic and sensory sources) or indirect vascular (vasoactive intestinal polypeptide VIP) influence to control lipid synthesis and/or excretion [2, 14, 15].

2.2 Aqueous component

The main non-reflex production of aqueous part of mucin/aqueous gel is from the Krauze and Wolfring glands (accessory lacrimal glands) located in the conjunctiva of superior eye lid and superior conjunctival fornix. The main lacrimal gland is responsible for aqueous tears production secondary to deleterious stimulation and plays important, though not entirely clear role in non-reflecting tearing (dry eye syndrome is noted in patients with damaged main lacrimal gland) [1, 7, 8, 11, 18]. The aqueous layer consists of water, electrolytes, proteins, cytokines, vitamins, immunoglobulins and peptide growth factors. Moreover, amino acids, bicarbonate, calcium, urea and magnesium were detected in tear film [15, 19].

The aqueous portion of the tear film is responsible for ocular surface lubrication, washing away foreign bodies or contaminations and nourishing avascular cornea (oxygen, inorganic salts, proteins, glucose) [3, 16, 20]. The soluble mucins decrease the surface tension, impact coherence of the aqueous layer, contribute to tear film viscosity [14, 19]. Almost 500 different proteins have been extracted from the tear film [3, 21]. Lactoferrin, lysozyme, lipocalin, secretory immunoglobulin A(sIgA), immunoglobulin G(IgG), immunoglobulin M (IgM), albumin, transferrin, ceruloplasmin, defensins, tear specific prealbumin and glycoproteins participate in the ocular surface antimicrobial activity and defense [3, 15, 22]. Growth factors, vitamins, electrolytes, neuropeptides and protease inhibitors are necessary for retaining ocular surface health and epithelial integrity [1, 3, 23]. Retinol, secreted by the lacrimal gland, is necessary for maintenance of goblet cells and regulates corneal epithelium desquamation, keratinization and metaplasia [15, 24–26].

The lacrimal gland is affected by both nervous system and various hormones [1, 2, 7, 11, 15, 18, 23, 27]. The gland innervation comes from the first brunch of trigeminal nerve, the facial nerve and sympathetic fibers from the superior cervical ganglion [1, 11, 15, 28]. Stimulation of the ocular surface is the beginning of the main lacrimal gland production (reflexing tearing). The emotional tearing is also connected with this reflex loop (**Figure 2**). The meaning of the sympathetic part of innervation is thought to stimulate basal tearing but is still not completely understood. The accessory lacrimal glands are heavily innervated, but there is lack of parasympathetic part and most of the innervation is undefined [8, 15, 29].

Androgens and estrogens influence lacrimal gland production. Androgens lack is responsible for reversible degenerative changes of lacrimal gland, decreased volume of the tears, decreased level of proteins in tears. Estrogens remain controversial: some studies described estrogen deficiency linked to keratoconjunctivitis sicca (KCS) and lacrimal gland degeneration, other works have shown no changes in the lacrimal gland and tear film with decreased level of estrogens [15, 17, 30, 31]. Thyroid stimulating hormone (TSH) receptors (present in lacrimal gland) as well as thyroid

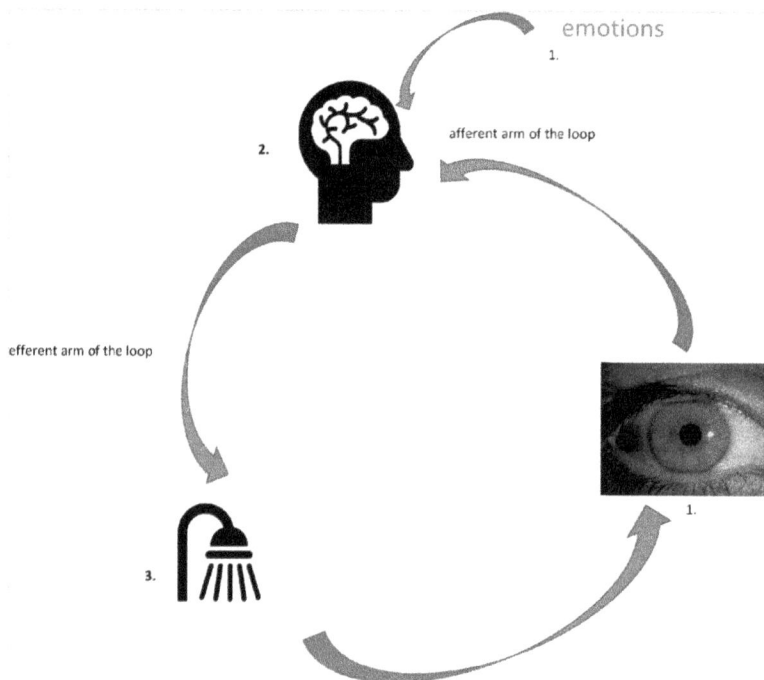

emotions
1.

afferent arm of the loop

2.

efferent arm of the loop

3.

1.

Figure 2.
Reflex loop of tearing: 1. Stimulants: - ocular surface and nasal mucosa - afferent arm of the loop (first branch of the fifth cranial nerve)- emotions, 2. brain - efferent arm of the loop (parasympathetic part of the seventh nerve), 3. lacrimal glands.

hormone and tissue interaction are necessary for lacrimal gland secretion. Adequate insulin level is important for lacrimal gland and ocular surface stability and function, because it is necessary for acinar cell and cornea epithelial cell proliferation [32].

2.3 Mucins

The mucous layer of the tear film is produced by both corneal and conjunctival epithelium and the lacrimal gland and conjunctival goblet cells [1, 3, 7, 11, 15, 33]. It is composed of secreted and transmembrane mucins, immunoglobulins, salts, urea, glucose, leukocytes, cellular debris and enzymes [1, 3, 15, 33–35].

Traditional description of the mucins role limits to secreted gel-forming mucins working as lubricating agents and clearing molecules. Current date indicate its role also as a barrier for corneal and conjunctival epithelium. We can find two kinds of the mucins: cell surface-associated and secreted [36].

Cell surface-associated mucins form a thick cell surface glycocalyx, providing through their O-glucans a disadhesive character to the apical surface of the corneal epithelium. That is why they assure boundary lubrication and prevent adhesion of corneal epithelium and tarsal conjunctiva during blinking and sleeping [36, 37]. Moreover, membrane-bound mucins take part in the maintenance of the mucosal barrier integrity to prevent the penetrance molecules onto ocular surface epithelia [36, 38]. Some recent studies have weighed up membrane-bound mucins as osmosensors in eukaryotic cells [36, 39, 40].

Secreted mucins have a capability to trap contaminations (e.g. allergens, debris, pathogens) in order to clearance them from mucosal surface. Gel-forming mucins retaining water, form highly hydrated gel to lubricate ocular surface and reduce shear stress during blinking or rubbing. Moreover, MUC 7 (detected in lacrimal gland), has potent antifungal and antimicrobial activity [34, 35, 37, 41–43].

Goblet cells may be stimulated for mucin secretion by histamine, antigen, immune complex, mechanical action (i.e. blinking), direct (muscarinic and α-adrenergic receptors on immature goblet cells) and indirect (sensory, sympathetic and parasympathetic innervation of conjunctiva surrounding goblet cells) neural control [15, 16, 44–46].

2.4 Tear film dynamics

Balanced tear film production and elimination is crucial for its integrity, stability and right osmolality [3]. Tear film production is a complex process, controlled by the various factors: main and accessory lacrimal glands, ocular surface structures (cornea, conjunctiva, eyelids with Meibomian gland) and interconnecting nerves (both sensory and motor) [3, 47, 48]. Ryc.1. Tears elimination proceeds as evaporation, drainage and absorption. Tear film interfaces with the environment; that is the reason of evaporation (about $1,4$–$39,3 \times 10^{-7}$ g/cm^2/s) [5, 49]. Some environmental factors like humidity, temperature and air movements impact the rate of tear evaporation from the ocular surface [50]. Higher evaporation is the reason of tear film thinning and, because of that, instability and hyperosmolality [51]. Regardless of the recent date on evaporation, tears outflow through the lacrimal drainage system remains the main way of its elimination. With each blink, tears with contaminations (like cellular debris, toxins, inflammatory cells and other waste products) are moved towards the lacrimal puncta and next - due to the negative pressure created in lacrimal drainage system - to the lacrimal drainage tract [3, 52]. Some studies noted reduction of tears production in patients with impaired drainage that highlights the importance of this process in the model of tear dynamics [53–55]. At least absorption: process necessary for proper tear film dynamics, connected with cornea, conjunctiva and - mainly - nasolacrimal duct epithelium [56]. The equilibrium in the tear film production, retention and elimination acts the crucial role in its proper functioning, thereby ocular surface health [3].

3. The influence of various diseases and conditions on the tear film

Tear film stability can be disturb in tear film layers deficiencies, defective spreading of the tear film, in some general diseases and during application of some general and/or topical medications. In the wake of it dry eye disease evolves [11, 36, 57] (**Tables 2** and **3**).

3.1 Lipid layer alteration

Deficiency of this layer is the reason of more rapid evaporation and in the absence of increased tear production activates evaporative form of dry eye disease [58].

The most common reason of lipid layer deficiency is obstruction of the Meibomian glands. Meibomian gland disfunction (MGD) may be provoked by various local and systemic conditions, e.g. atopic keratoconjunctivitis, chronic blepharitis [59, 60], generalized dysfunction of sebaceous glands (rosacea, seborrheic dermatitis), chemical agents such as turpentine, present in the sick building environment [36, 61]. Tobacco smokers are prone to development of MGD [62], the more severe course of MGD was observed in type 2 diabetes mellitus [63].

Dry eye	
Aqueous deficient dry eye (ADDE)	Evaporative dry eye (EDE)

Sjőgren syndrome dry eye (SSDE)
   Primary
   Secondary
	Endogenous
	   Meibomian gland dysfunction (MGD)
	   Disorders of lids and lid aperture
	   Low blinking
	   Systemic medicines

Non- Sjőgren Syndrome dry eye
   Lacrimal deficiency
   Lacrimal gland duct obstruction
   Reflex block
   Systemic medicines
	Exogenous
	   Contact lens wear
	   Ocular surface diseases
	   Topical medicines
	   Vitamin A deficiency

Table 2.
Dry eye classification [7, 23, 64–74].

Dry eye disease	
Signs	Symptoms
• Discomfort: itching, stinging, burning, "foreign body sensation" occasionally pain, photophobia • Visual fluctuations (especially during reading- blinking recover vision) • Tear film instability (potential damage of ocular surface)	• Eyelids: blepharitis posterior, Meibomian gland disfunction, trichiasis, symblepharon • Conjunctiva: hyperemia, keratonization, persistent inflammation, dyeing with the lissamine green(rose bengal) • Tear film: debris, reduced meniscus, instability(reduced break-up time), elevated osmolarity and level of inflammatory mediators • Cornea: epithelial defect (dyeing with the fluorescein), filaments, mucus clumping • Potential complications: persistent epithelial defect, keratomalacia, corneal perforation, corneal ulcer

Table 3.
Signs and symptoms of dry eye disease [1, 7, 23, 64].

Furthermore, the insufficient protein intake in bariatric patients negatively influences tear film lipids [75]. Also androgen deficiency (e.g. aging, anti-androgen therapy, congenital impairment or absence of the androgen receptor) hinders lipid production [76]. Incomplete blinking has been reported as the reason for lipid layer instability, because of inadequate lipid distribution [9, 77]. Some studies have revealed influence of medicines on the lipid layer: e.g. isotretinoin decreases Meibomian gland secretory ability [78], and on the contrary, botulinum neurotoxin A injections seem to increase lipid layer thickness [79].

3.2 Aqueous layer disturbances

Aqueous layer deficiency is the most common reason of dry eye and is classified into two groups: Sjögren Syndrome dry eye and non-Sjögren Syndrome dry eye [64, 65].

Sjögren's syndrome (SS) is a rheumatic autoimmune disease in which exocrine glands (salivary and lacrimal glands) are involved that results in clinical symptoms of dry mouth and dry eye. SS can be primary-pSS (without any other accompanying symptoms) or secondary-sSS (with other autoimmune diseases: systemic lupus erythematosus (SLE), rheumatoid arthritis (RA), polyarteritis nodosa, systemic sclerosis, granulomatosis with polyangiitis (GPA), primary biliary cholangitis (PBC), mixed connective tissue disease, occult thyroid eye disease) [64, 66]. Some studies demonstrated coincidence of dry eye disease (DED) and SS in 46.7% cases [64, 67].

In non-SS dry eye reduced tear secretion is a result of senile hyposecretion, lacrimal excision, lacrimal duct obstruction, immune lacrimal gland damage in sarcoidosis or lymphoma, sensory or motor reflex block, scarring conditions of the conjunctiva (pemphigoid, chemical burns, trachoma, chronic ocular Graft-versus-Host Disease) [11, 57, 64, 68, 69]. Corneal hypoesthesia and due to it dry eye can be result of corneal refraction surgery [70], contact lens wearing [71], herpetic keratitis or as a side effect after surgical trigeminal neuralgia management [72].

Increased electrolyte concentration, loss of growth factors, presence of proinflammatory cytokines result in changes in composition of the aqueous part of the tear film. Such a disturbances in connection with slow tear turnover are secondary to ocular surface damage [8, 47].

There are some medicines reported to exacerbate tear secretion, e.g. thiazide diuretics, tricyclic and tetracyclic antidepressants, ß-blokers, anticholinergics, benzodiazepines, antihistamines, antihypertensives and anti-Parkinson's drugs [8, 57, 73, 74].

3.3 Mucin layer deficiency

Disturbances of the mucin layer are connected with the goblet cell deficiency, which is observed in majority forms of dry eye [8, 80]. The leading reason of xerophthalmia connected with mucins the insufficiency of vitamin A is [8, 57, 81, 82]. The lack of vitamin A is usually connected with various forms of malnutrition or chronic malabsorption. Gastroenterological diseases (e.g. coeliac disease) impair vitamin A absorption [83–85]. Conditions affecting liver impair fat metabolism and decreases absorption of this fat-soluble vitamin [86, 87]. Pancreas insufficiency (e.g. cystic fibrosis) hinders vitamin A intake by its influence on fat digestion pathway [88, 89]. Alcoholism, restrictive diets (both in eating disorders and selective, like poor balanced vegans') and low-quality food consumption are the most common reasons of malnutrition and because of that vitamin A insufficiency [90–94].

There are some problems responsible for impairment of goblet cells function. Mucous membrane pemphigoid and its subtype – ocular cicatricial pemphigoid via recurrent inflammation destroy goblet cells and promote subepithelial fibrosis, resulting in changes ranging from xerophthalmia to conjunctival keratinization and blindness [95–99]. Stevens-Johnson Syndrome, trachoma and severe burns (both thermal and chemical) impair mucin production by decreasing the number of active goblet cells [8, 100–103].

Moreover, some medications (e.g. mucolytics, antihistamines) and preservatives influence the ocular surface and modify mucous layer [8, 57, 104].

3.4 Multilayer disturbances

Although three layers of the tear film are investigated, all of them remain in strict dependence of each other and many conditions cause disturbances of the tear film as a whole. The most common problem impairing ocular surface is progression with age; decreased tear production, tantalic problems, hormonal changes, medications and other diseases affect tear production, its' ingredients and spreading over the ocular surface [8, 57, 105, 106]. Tantalic dry eye seems to be one of the most important conditions influencing all three layers: eyelid incongruency (entropion, ectropion, lid margin irregularities, exophthalmos), epitheliopathy (e.g. corneal scars) and evaporation are the reason of tear loss. Neurological problems (both afferent and efferent part of the reflex loop) directly affect tear secretion [8, 57, 105].

Hormonal changes (androgens, estrogens, prolactin, thyroid hormone, insulin resistance/deprivation, ACTH resistance, adrenal insufficiency, multiple endocrine deficiency) influence tear stability as well [105, 106]. Meanwhile, the newest meta-analysis revealed no correlation between hormonal replacement therapy or oral contraceptives and tear film – it seems to be speculative [107, 108]. Dry eye disease due to hormonal disorders often connect both aqueous tear deficient and evaporative mechanism. Thyroid associated diseases result usually in autoimmune condition (impaired thyroid hormone activity, autoantibodies against THS receptors present in lacrimal glands, autoantibodies against thyroid hormone and/or their receptors) but the final effect of dry eye is connected also with ocular surface disturbances due to enhanced environment exposure, lid mechanical impairment (reduced lipids secretion, eyelid retraction, eye globe proptosis, impaired blinking) and therapy (thyroid hormone replacement, iodine suppression, immunomodulators specific for orbit and ocular disease, local radiotherapy and surgical procedures) [106]. In patients with diabetes mellitus the frequency of dryness varies from 15.4 to 82%. The mechanism of dry eye disease in diabetic patients is multifactorial: insulin resistance or deprivation is responsible for lacrimal gland size reduction, histological and molecular changes of it, polyneuropathy and nerve-conduction abnormalities that reduce secretion. Peripheral microvascular disease and insulin reduced input in target tissues are the other reasons of lacrimal gland and ocular surface disorders. Tear film instability and higher osmolarity are probably the result of higher glucose and protein levels in the tears and changes in the protein profile [106, 109].

In literature there are examples of dry eye disease secondary to other hormonal imbalance (e.g. ACTH-triple A syndrome, multiple endocrine deficiency) [106, 110].

Some environmental factors (e.g. pollutions, visual display terminals, temperature, humidity) promotes dry eye disease, however the pathomechanism is still discussed [111, 112]. Contact lenses wear influences lipid layer, changes the dynamics of the whole tear film and is the reason of dry eye symptoms [113–115].

There are a lot of date on the influence of medications (both topical and systemic) on the tear film. Some samples: ß-blockers used for glaucoma therapy reduce test Shirmer I and break-up time values, long term general anesthesia decrease basal tear production, antihistamines block both goblet cells and lacrimal glands, topical glaucoma therapy reduces LLT, oral mucolytics modify mucous layer, systemic

	Causes of disturbances
Lipid layer	MGD: atopic local changes, chronic blepharitis, generalized dysfunction of the sebaceous glands, chemical agents, tabacco smokers, diabetes mellitus Insufficient protein intake (bariatric patients) Androgen deficiency: aging, anti-androgen therapy, congenital impairment or absence of the androgen receptor Incomplete blinking (inadequate lipid distribution) Medicins
Aqueous layer	• Sjőgren syndrome dry eye (SSDE) (primary, without other accompanying symptoms and secondary, with other autoimmune diseases) • Non- Sjőgren syndrome dry eye (nSSDE) (senile hyposecretion, lacrimal excision, lacrimal duct obstruction, immune lacrimal gland damage, sensor or motor reflex block, scarring condition of the conjunctiva, corneal hypoesthesia as a result of CL wearing, heretical keratitis or surgical procedures) • Medicines
Mucus layer	• Insufficiency of vitamin A: malnutrition or malabsorption (gastroenterological diseases, condition affecting liver, pancreas insufficiency, alcoholism, restrictive diets, low quality food) • Destruction of the goblet cells (cicatricial conjunctival changes: e.g. pemphigoid, Stevens-Johnson syndrome, trachoma, GVHD, severe thermal and chemical burns) • Medicines
Multilayer	• Aging: decreased tear production, tantalic problems (eyelid incongruency as entropion, ectropion, eyelid irregularities, exophthalmos, epitheliopathy; e.g. corneal scars) • Hormonal changes (androgens, estrogens, prolactin, ACTH, thyroid hormone) • Neurological problems (both afferent and efferent part of the reflex loop) • Environment (pollutions, ambient temperature, humidity) • Visual display terminals • Medicines (both topical and systemic) • Preservatives

Table 4.
The main causes of tear film deficiency [7, 58–125].

antidepressants, anticholinergics or antihypertensives increase risk of dry eye problems [56, 103, 116–122]. A comprehensive review of this problem with the list of medicines and herbs has been prepared by Askeroglu et al. [123]. Analyzing influence of medicines on the ocular surface and dry eye disease we have to remember that topical used multidose artificial tears and lubricants contain preservatives. The most common Benzalkonium chloride – BAK disrupts tear stability, causes corneal and conjunctival epithelium damage and induces inflammatory changes that depends on dose and time of use. Alternative preservatives (e.g. Polyquaternium-I: Polyquad®, Polyhexamethylene biguanide: PHMB, Sodium perborate: GenAqua®, Deqest®, stabilized Oxychlorocomplex SOC: Purite®, OcuPure®, ionic-buffered solution containing zinc chloride, borate, propylate glucol and sorbitol:Sofzia) are used in some artificial tears, lubricants or glaucoma drops. Published date on the ocular performance of them generally show they induce significantly less disturbances of the ocular surface than BAK [124, 125] (**Table 4**).

4. Conclusions

The ocular surface contacts with the environment by the tear film as interface. Thus, tear production, composition, dynamics and function is so important to prevent it healthy. There are many diseases and conditions (both systemic and local) that may affect each layer of the tear film separately or all of them together. Moreover, tear film disorders can manifest systemic diseases and, sometimes, be necessary or even be the only clue to diagnosis. The commonness of tear film problems and wide spectrum of its different background seem to require to be considered in everyday medical, not only ophthalmological, practice. Those problems should be analyzed to plan and undertake proper therapy, especially in patients with eye dryness symptoms.

Author details

Dorota Kopacz[1,2*], Łucja Niezgoda[1], Ewa Fudalej[1], Anna Nowak[1] and Piotr Maciejewicz[1,2]

1 Medical University of Warsaw, Warsaw, Poland

2 Department of Ophthalmology, Infant Jesus Teaching Hospital, Warsaw, Poland

*Address all correspondence to: dr.dk@wp.pl

IntechOpen

References

[1] Holland EJ, Mannis MJ, Lee WB: Ocular Surface Diseases, Elseviere Inc, 2013

[2] Dartt DA, Willcox MDP; Complexity of the tear film: importance in homeostasis and dysfunction during disease. Exp Eye Res 2013, December,117:1-3

[3] Stahl U, Willcox M, Stapleton F; Osmolality and tear film dynamics. Clin Exp Optom 2012, 95(1):3-11

[4] de Paiva CS, Pflugfelder SC; Tera clearance implications for ocular surface health. Ex Eye Res 2004, 78:395-397

[5] Mathers W; Evaporation from the ocular surface. Exp Eye Res 2004, 78:389-394

[6] Tiffany JM. The normal tear film. Dev Ophthalmol 2008, 41:1-20

[7] Willcox MDP, Argüeso P, Georgiev GA, Holopainen JM, Laurie GW, Millar TJ, Papas EB, Rolland JP, Schmidt TA, Stahl U, Suarez T, Subbaraman LN, Uçakhan OO, MDk, Jones L; TFOS DEWS II Tear Film Report. Ocul Surf. 2017 July ; 15(3): 366-403. doi:10.1016/j.jtos.2017.03.006.

[8] Rolando M, Zierhut M; The ocular surface and tear film and their dysfunction in dry eye disease. Surv Ophthalmol 2001, 45(supl2):S203-210

[9] Yokoi, N., A.J. Bron, and G.A. Georgiev, The precorneal tear film as a fluid shell: the effect of blinking and saccades on tear film distribution and dynamics. Ocul Surf 2014, 12(4):252-266.

[10] McCulley JP, Shine WA; A compositional based model for the tear film lipid layer. Trans Am Ophthalmol Soc 1997. 95:79-88

[11] Daily PM. Structure and function of the tear film. Adv Exp Med Biol 1994, 350:239-247

[12] Bron A, Tiffany JM, Gouveia S, Yokoi N, Voon L; Functional aspects of the tear film lipid layer. Exp Eye Res 2004, 78:347-360

[13] Foulks GN; The correlation between the tear film lipid layer and dry eye disease. Surv Ophthalmol 2007, 52(4):369-374

[14] McCulley JP, Shine WE; The lipid layer of tears: dependent on Meibomian gland function. Exp Eye Res 2004, 78:361-365

[15] Davidson HJ, Kuonen VJ; The tear film and ocular mucins. Vet Ophthalmology 2004, 7(2):71-77

[16] Dartt DA; Regulation of tear secration. Adv Exp Med Biol 1994, 350:1-10

[17] Sullivan DA, Sullivan BD, Ulman MD, Rocha EM, Krenzer KL, Cermak JM, Toda I, Doane MG, Evans JE, Wickham LA.: Androgen influence of the Meibomian gland. Invest Ophthalmol Vis Sci 2000, 41(12): 3732-3742

[18] Conardy CD, Joos ZP, Patel BCK; Review: The lacrimal gland and its role in dry eye. J Ophthalmol 2016, 2016:7542929, doi: 10.1155/2016/7542929. Epub 2016 Mar 2.

[19] Iwata S; Chemical composition of the aqueous phase. Int Ophthalmol Clin Spring 1973;13(1):29-46.doi: 10.1097/00004397-197301310-00005.

[20] Kaura R, Tiffany JM; The role of mucous glykoproteins in the tear film. in: Holly FJ: The preocular tear film in health, disease and contact lens wear.

Dry Eye Institute Inc, Lubbock, 1986:728-731

[21] de Souza GA, Godoy LM, Mann M; Identification of 491 proteins in the tear film proteome reveals a large number of proteases protease inhibitors. Genome Biol 2006, 7:R72

[22] Huang LC, Jean D, Proske RJ, Reins RY, McDermott AM; Ocular surface expression and in vitro activity of antimicrobial peptides. Curr Eye Res 2007, 32:595-609

[23] Lemp MA, Beuerman RW; Tear film. in Krachmer JH, Mannis MJ, Holland EJ: Cornea. Elsevier Inc, 2011:33-39

[24] Ubels JL, Foley KM, Rismondo V. Retinol secretion by the lacrimal gland. Invest Ophthalmol Vis Sci. 1986 Aug;27(8):1261-8.

[25] Ubels JL, Rismondo V, Osgood TB; The Relationship Between Secretion of Retinol and Protein by the Lacrimal Gland. Invest Ophthalmol Vis Sci 1989, 30(5):952-960

[26] Pfister RR, Renner ME; The corneal and conjunctival surface in vitamin A deficiency: a scanning electron microscopy study. Invest Ophthalmol Vis Sci 1978, 17(9): 874-883

[27] Obata H; Anatomy and histopathology of the human lacrimal gland. Cornea 2006, 25 (10) (Supl.1):S82-S89

[28] American Academy of Ophthalmology; Orbit, eyelids and lacrimal system. In Basic and Clinical Science Course 1998-1999

[29] Riley CM, Day RC, Greeley DM, Langford WS; Central automatic dysfunction with defective lacrimation; report of five cases. Pediatrics 1949, 3(4):468-478

[30] Sullivan DA, Kelleher RS, Vaerman JP, Hann LE; Androgen regulation of secretory component synthesis by lacrimal gland acinar cells in vitro. J Immunol 1990, 145:4238-4244

[31] Sullivan DA, Wickham LA, Rocha EM, Kelleher RS, da Silveira LA, Toda I; Influence of gender, sex steroid hormones and the hypothalamic-pituitary axis on the structure and function of the lacrimal gland. Adv Exp Med Biol 1998, 438:11-42

[32] Rocha EM, Mantelli F, Nominato LF, Bonini S; Hormones and dry eye syndrome:an update on what we do and don't know. Curr Opin Ophthalmol 2013, 24:348-355Gipson IK, 33. Inatomi T; Cellular origin of mucins of ocular surface tear film. Adv Exp Med Biol 1998, 4(38):221-227

[33] Gipson IK, Argueso P; Role of mucins in the function of the corneal and conjunctival epithelia. Int Rev Cytol 2003, 231:1-46

[34] Gipson IK; Distribution of mucins at the ocular surface. Exp Eye Res 2004, 78:379-388

[35] Nichols BA, Chiappino ML, Dawson CR. Demonstration of the mucous layer of the tear film by electron microscopy. Invest Ophthalmol Vis Sci 1985, 26:464-473

[36] Mantelli F, Argueso P; Functions of ocular surface mucins in health and disease. Curr Opin Allergy Clin Immunol 2008, 8(5):477-483

[37] Sumiyoshi M, Ricciuto J Tisdale A, Gipson IA, Mantelli F, Argueso P; Antiadhesive character of mucin O-glycans confer an surface of the corneal epithelial cells. Invest Ophthalmol Vis Sci 2008,49:197-203

[38] Argueso P, Tisdale A, Spurr-Michaud S, Sumiyoshi M, Gipson IK; Mucin characteristics of human

corneal-limbal epithelial cell that exclude the rose Bengal anionic dye. Invest Ophthalmol Vis Sci 2006, 47:113-119

[39] Tatebayashi K, Tanaka K, Yang HY, Yamamoto K, Matsushita Y, Tomida T, Imai M, Saito H; Transmembrane mucins Hrk1 and Msb 2 are putative osmosensors in the SHO 1 branch of yeast HOG pathway. EMBO J 2007,26:3521-3533

[40] De Nadal E, Real FX, Posas F; Mucins , osmosensors in eukaryotic cells? Trends Cell Biol 2007, 17:571-574

[41] McKenzie RW, Jumblatt JE, Jumblatt MM; Quantification of MUC2 and MUC5AC transcripts in human conjunctiva. Invest Ophthalmol Vis Sci 2000, 41:703-708

[42] Dilly PN; Conjunctival cells, subsurface vesicles and tear film mucus. in: Holly FJ: The preocular tear film in health, disease and contact lens wear. Dry Eye Institute Inc, Lubbock, 1986:677-687

[43] Chandler JW, Gillette TE; Immunologic defense mechanisms of the ocular surface. Ophthalmol 1983, 90:585-591

[44] Bobek LA, Situ H; MUC7 20-mer: investigation of microbial activity, secondary structure and possible mechanism of antifungal action. Antimicrob Agents Chemometer 2003,47:643-652

[45] Dartt DA, McCarthy DM, Mercer HJ, Kessler TL, Chung EH, Zieske JD; Localization of nerves adjacent to goblet cells in rat conjunctiva. Curr Eye Res 1995, 14:993-1000

[46] Rios JD, Forde K, Diebold Y, Lightman J, Zieske JD, Dartt DA; Development of conjunctival goblet cells and their neuroreceptor subtype expression. Invest Ophthalmol Med Sci 2000, 41:2127-2137

[47] Stern MF, Bauerman RW, Fox RI, Gao J, Mircheff AK, Pflugfelder SC; the pathology of dry eye :the interaction between the ocular surface and lacrimal glands. Cornea 1998, 17:584-589

[48] Stern ME, Gao J, Siemasko KF, Bauerman RW, Pflugfelder SC; The role of the lacrimal functional unit in the pathology of dry eye. Exp Eye Res 2004, 78:409-416

[49] Tomlinson A; inputs and outputs of the lacrimal system: review of production and evaporative loss. Ocul Surf 2009,7:186-198

[50] Borchman D, Foulks GN, Yappert MC, Mathews J, Leake K, Bell J; Factors affecting evaporation rates of the tear film components measured in vitro. Eye Contac Lens 2009, 35:32-37

[51] King-Smith PE, Nichols JJ, Nichols KK, Fink BA, Braun RJ; Contributions of evaporation and other mechanisms to tear film thinning and break-up. Optom Vis Sci 2008, 85:623-630

[52] Lemp MA, Weiler HH; How do tears exit? Invest Ophthalmol Vis Sci 1983, 24:619-622

[53] Francois J, Neetens A; Tear flow in man. Am J Ophthalmol 1973, 76:351-358

[54] Yen MT, Pflugfelder SC, Feuer WJ; The effect of punctal occlusion on tear production, tear clearance and ocular surface sensation in normal subjects. Am J Ophthalmol 2001, 131:314-323

[55] Stahl U, Francis IC, Stapleton F; Prospective controlled study of vapor pressure tear osmolality and tear meniscus height in nasolacrimal duct obstruction. Am J Ophthalmol 2006, 141:1051-1056

[56] Tomlinson A, Khanal S; Assessment of Tear Film Dynamics: Quantification Approach. Ocul Surf 2005 Apr;3(2):81-95.

[57] Niezgoda Ł, Fudalej E, Nowak A, Kopacz D; Tear film disorders as a manifestation of various diseases and conditions. Klinika Oczna 2020, article in press.

[58] Rolando M, Refojo MF, Kenyon KR; Tear water evaporation and eye surface diseases. Ophthalmologica 1985, 190:147-149

[59] Mathers WD, Lane JA; Meibomian gland lipids, evaporation and tear film stability. Adv Exp Med Biol 1998, 438:349-360

[60] Shine WE, McCulley JP; Meibomian gland triglyceride fatty acid differences in chronic blepharitis patients. Cornea 1996, 15(4):340-346

[61] Franck C, Bach E, Skov P. Prevalence of objective eye manifestations in people working in office buildings with different prevalences of the sick building syndrome compared with the general population. Int Arch Occup Environ Health. 1993;65(1):65-69

[62] Altinors DD, Akça S, Akova YA, Bilezikçi B, Goto E, Dogru M, Tsubota K; Smoking associated with damage to the lipid layer of the ocular surface. Am J Ophthalmol. 2006 Jun;141(6):1016-1021.

[63] Sandra Johanna GP, Antonio LA, Andrés GS. Correlation between type 2 diabetes, dry eye and Meibomian glands dysfunction. J Optom. 2019;12(4):256-262.

[64] Kopacz D, Maciejewicz P; Sjögren's Syndrome as an Ocular Problem: Signs and Symptoms, Diagnosis, Treatment. In: Maślińska M; Chronic Autoimmune Epithelitis – Sjogren's Syndrome and other Autoimmune Diseases of the Exocrine Glands. IntechOpen 2019

[65] Lin H, Yiu SC; Dry eye disease: A review of diagnostic approaches and treatment. Saudi J Ophthalmol 2014, 28(3):173-181

[66] Voulgarelis M, Tzioufas AG. Current Aspects of Pathogenesis in Sjögren's Syndrome. Ther Adv Musculoskelet Dis. 2010,2(6):325-334

[67] Ken E, Demirag MD, Beyazyildz E. Presence of Sjogren's syndrome in dry eye patients. Rheumatology (Sunnyvale) 2014,4(2):137

[68] Craig JP, Nichols KK, Akpek EK, Caffery B, Dua HS, Joo CK, et al. TFOS DEWS II Definition and Classification Report. Ocul Surf. 2017;15(3):276-8

[69] Kopacz D, Maciejewicz P; Objawy okulistyczne w przebiegu choroby „przeszczep przeciwko gospodarzowi" po allogenicznym przeszczepie komórek macierzystych szpiku/ Ocular Manifestation of Graft-Versus-Host Disease Following Allogenic Hematopoietic Stem Cells Transplantation. Okulistyka 2/2016:35-37

[70] Bragheeth MA, Dua HS. Corneal sensation after myopic and hyperopic LASIK: clinical and confocal microscopic study. Br J Ophthalmol. 2005;89(5):580-585

[71] Murphy PJ, Patel S, Marshall J. The effect of long-term, daily contact lens wear on corneal sensitivity. Cornea. 2001;20(3):264-269

[72] Semeraro F, Forbice E, Romano V, et al. Neurotrophic keratitis. Ophthalmologica. 2014;231(4):191-197

[73] Koçer E, Koçer A, Özsütçü M, Dursun AE, Krpnar İ. Dry Eye Related to Commonly Used New Antidepressants. J Clin Psychopharmacol. 2015;35(4):411-413

[74] Bergmann MT, Newman BL, Johnson NC, Jr. The effect of a

diuretic (hydrochlorothiazide) on tear production in humans. Am J Ophthalmol. 1985;99(4):473-475

[75] Sánchez-Sánchez AS, Rodríguez-Murguía N, Martinez-Cordero C, Chávez-Cerda S. Protein Diet in Bariatric Patients Could Modify Tear Film. Obes Surg. 2020;30(5):2053-2055.

[76] Krenzer KL, Dana MR, Ullman MD, et al. Effect of androgen deficiency on the human meibomian gland and ocular surface. J Clin Endocrinol Metab. 2000;85(12):4874-4882

[77] Wang MTM, Tien L, Han A, et al. Impact of blinking on ocular surface and tear film parameters. Ocul Surf. 2018;16(4):424-429

[78] Moy A, McNamara, LinMC; Effect of isotretoinin on meibomian glands. Optom Vis Sci 2015, 92(9):925-930

[79] Ho RW, Fang PC, Chao TL, Chien CC, Kuo MT. Increase lipid tear thickness after botulinum neurotoxin A injection in patients with blepharospasm and hemifacial spasm. Sci Rep. 2018;8(1):8367

[80] Sommer A, Emran N; Tear production in vitamin A-responsive xerophthalmia. Am J Ophthalmol 1982, 93:84-87

[81] Wiseman EM, Bar-El Dadon S, Reifen R. The vicious cycle of vitamin a deficiency: A review. Crit Rev Food Sci Nutr. 2017, 57(17):3703-3714.

[82] Whatham A, Bartlett H, Eperjesi F, Blumenthal C, Allen J, Suttle C, Gaskin K; Vitamin and mineral deficiencies in the developed world and their effect on the eye and vision. Ophthalmic Physiol Opt. 2008, 28(1):1-12

[83] Chiu M, Dillon A, Watson S. Vitamin A deficiency and xerophthalmia in children of a developed country. J Paediatr Child Health. 2016, 52(7):699-703.

[84] da Cruz SP, Matos A, Pereira S, Saboya C, da Cruz SP, Ramalho A. Roux-en-Y; Gastric Bypass Aggravates Vitamin A Deficiency in the Mother-Child Group. Obes Surg. 2018, 28(1):114-121.

[85] Cheshire J, Kolli ; Vitamin A deficiency due to chronic malabsorption: an ophthalmic manifestation of a systemic condition. BMJ Case Rep. 2017;2017, doi: 10.1136/bcr-2017-220024corr1

[86] Kemp CM, Jacobson SG, Faulkner DJ, Walt RW; Visual function and rhodopsin levels in humans with vitamin A deficiency. Exp Eye Res. 1988, 46(2):185-197.

[87] Prasad D, Bhriguvanshi A; Ocular manifestations of liver disease in children: Clinical aspects and implications. Ann Hepatol. 2019. S1665-2681(19)32293-8. doi:10.1016/j.aohep.2019.11.009

[88] Morkeberg JC, Edmund C, Prause JU, Lanng S, Koch C, Michaelsen KF; Ocular findings in cystic fibrosis patients receiving vitamin A supplementation. Graefes Arch Clin Exp Ophthalmol. 1995, 233(11):709-13.

[89] Norsa L, Zazzeron L, Cuomo M, Claut L, Bulfamante AMC, Biffi A, Colombo C; Night Blindness in Cystic Fibrosis: The Key Role of Vitamin A in the Digestive System. Nutrients. 2019;11(8) :1876. doi:10.3390/nu11081876

[90] Roncone DP; Xerophthalmia secondary to alcohol-induced malnutrition. Optometry. 2006, 77(3):124-133.

[91] Kopecky A, Benda F, Nemcansky J; Xerosis in Patient with Vitamin A

Deficiency - a Case Report. Cesk Slov Oftalmol. 2018, 73(5-6):222-224.

[92] Martini S, Rizzello A, Corsini I, Romanin B, Fiorentino M, Grandi S, Bergamashi S; Vitamin A Deficiency Due to Selective Eating as a Cause of Blindness in a High-Income Setting. Pediatrics. 2018, 141(Suppl 5):S439-S444.

[93] Jaworowski S, Drabkin E, Rozenman Y; Xerophthalmia and undiagnosed eating disorder. Psychosomatics. 2002, 43(6):506-507.

[94] Kirby M, Danner E; Nutritional deficiencies in children on restricted diets. Pediatr Clin North Am. 2009, 56(5):1085-1103.

[95] Chan LS; Ocular and oral mucous membrane pemphigoid (cicatricial pemphigoid). Clin Dermatol. 2012, 30(1):34-37.

[96] Saw VP, Dart JK; Ocular mucous membrane pemphigoid: diagnosis and management strategies. Ocul Surf. 2008, 6(3):128-142.

[97] Ahmed M, Zein G, Khawaja F, Foster CS; Ocular cicatricial pemphigoid: pathogenesis, diagnosis and treatment. Prog Retin Eye Res. 2004, 23(6):579-592.

[98] Queisi MM, Zein M, Lamba N, Meese H, Foster CS; Update on ocular cicatricial pemphigoid and emerging treatments. Surv Ophthalmol. 2016,61(3):314-317.

[99] Kopacz D, Maciejewicz P, Kęcik D; Postać oczna pemfigoidu bliznowaciejącego – patogeneza i leczenie/ Ocular Mucous Membrane Pemphigoid – Pathogenesis and Treatment. Okulistyka 2/2016:7-9

[100] Arstikaitis MJ; Ocular aftermath of Stevens-Johnson syndrome. Arch Ophthalmol. 1973;90(5):376-379.

[101] Ralph RA; Conjunctival goblet cell density in normal subjects and in dry eye syndromes. Invest Ophthalmol. 1975,14(4):299-302.

[102] Wright P, Collin JR; The ocular complications of erythema multiforme (Stevens Johnson syndrome) and their management. Trans Ophthalmol Soc U K.1983,103(Pt 3):338-341.

[103] Lin A, Patel N, Yoo D, DeMartelaere S, Bouchard C; Management of ocular conditions in the burn unit: thermal and chemical burns and Stevens-Johnson syndrome/toxic epidermal necrolysis. J Burn Care Res. 2011, 32(5):547-560.

[104] Kim D, Kim HJ, Hyon JY, Wee WR, Shin YJ. Effects of oral mucolytics on tear film and ocular surface. Cornea. 2013, 32(7):933-938.

[105] Murube J, Nemeth J, Hoh H, Kaynak-Hekimhan P, Horwath-Winter J, Agarwal A, Baudouin C, Benítez del Castillo JM, Cervenka S, ChenZhuo L, Ducasse A, Durán J, Holly F, Javate R, Nepp J, Paulsen F, Rahimi A, Raus P, Shalaby O, Sieg P, Soriano H, Spinelli D, Ugurbas SH, Van Setten G; The triple classification of dry eye for practical clinical use. Eur J Ophthalmol. 2005, 15(6):660-667.

[106] Truong S, Cole N, Stapleton F, Golebiowski B. Sex hormones and the dry eye; Clin Exp Optom. 2014, 97(4):324-336.

[107] Dang A, Nayeni M, Mather R, Malvankar-Mehta MS; Hormone replacement therapy for dry eye disease patients: systematic review and meta-analysis. Can J Ophthalmol. 2020, 55(1):3-11.

[108] Moschos MM, Nitoda E.; The impact of combined oral contraceptives on ocular tissues: a review of ocular effects. Int J Ophthalmol. 2017, 10(10):1604-1610.

[109] Modulo CM, Jorge AG, Dias AC; Influence of insulin treatment on the lacrimal gland and ocular surfaceof diabetic rats. Endocrine 2009, 36:161-168

[110] Alves M, Dias AC, Rocha EM; Dry eye in childhood: epidemiological and clinical aspects. Ocul Surf 2008, 6:44-51

[111] Courtin R, Pereira B, Naughton G, Chamoux A, Chiambaretta F, Lanhers C, Dutheil F; Prevalence of dry eye disease in visual display terminal workers: a systematic review and meta-analysis. BMJ Open. 2016, 6(1):e009675.

[112] Hanyuda A, Sawada N, Uchino M, Kawashima M, Yuki K, Tsubota K, Yamagishi K, Iso H, Yasuda N, Saito I, Kato T, Abe Y, Arima K, Tanno K, Sakata K, Shimazu T, Yamaji T, Goto A, Inoue M, Iwasaki M, Tsugan S; Physical inactivity, prolonged sedentary behaviors, and use of visual display terminals as potential risk factors for dry eye disease: JPHC-NEXT study. Ocul Surf. 2020, 18(1):56-63.

[113] Mann A, Tighe B. Contact lens interactions with the tear film; Exp Eye Res. 2013, 117:88-98.

[114] Lim CHL, Stapleton F, Mehta JS.; Review of Contact Lens-Related Complications. Eye Contact Lens. 2018, 44 Suppl 2:S1-S10.

[115] Alipour F, Khaheshi S, Soleimanzadeh M, Heidarzadeh S, Heydarzadeh S; Contact Lens-related Complications: A Review. J Ophthalmic Vis Res. 2017, 12(2):193-204.

[116] Ohtsuki M, Yokoi N, Mori K, Matsumoto Y, Adachi W, Ishibashi K, Sato M, Kinoshita S;[Adverse effects of beta-blocker eye drops on the ocular surface]. Nippon Ganka Gakkai Zasshi. 2001, 105(3):149-154.

[117] Nielsen NV, Eriksen JS; Timolol transitory manifestations of dry eyes in long term treatment. Acta Ophthalmol (Copenh). 1979, 57(3):418-424.

[118] Lee SM, Lee JE, Kim SI, Jung JH, Shin J; Effect of topical glaucoma medication on tear lipid layer thickness in patients with unilateral glaucoma. Indian J Ophthalmol. 2019, 67(8):1297-302.

[119] Zernii EY, Golovastova MO, Baksheeva VE, Kabanova EI, Ishutina IE, Gancharova OS, Gusev AE, SavchenkoMS, Loboda AP, SotnikovaLA, Zamyatnin Jr AA, Philippov PP, Senin II; Alterations in Tear Biochemistry Associated with Postanesthetic Chronic Dry Eye Syndrome. Biochemistry (Mosc). 2016, 81(12):1549-57.

[120] Bielory L; Ocular toxicity of systemic asthma and allergy treatments. Curr Allergy Asthma Rep. 2006, 6(4):299-305.

[121] Norn M; The effect of drugs on tear flow. Trans Ophthalmol SOc UK 1985, 104:410-414.

[122] Sraux F, Martin P, Morax S, Offert H; Hyposecretion lacrimale et medicaments psychotropes. Ann Ocl 1976, 209:193-197

[123] Askeroglu U, Alleyne B, Guyuron B; Pharmaceutical and herbal products that may contribute to dry eyes. Plast Reconstr Surg. 2013, 131(1):159-167

[124] Maciejewicz P, Kopacz D; Substancje pomocnicze zawarte w kroplach do oczu/The Pharmaceutical Excipients Commonly Used in Eye Drops. Okulistyka 2016, 1:33-36

[125] Walsh K, Jones L. The use of preservatives in dry eye drops. *Clin Ophthalmol*. 2019;13:1409-1425.

Chapter 2

Biofilm Theory for Lid Margin and Dry Eye Disease

Maria Vincent, Jose Quintero, Henry D. Perry
and James M. Rynerson

Abstract

Blepharitis and dry eye disease have long been viewed as two distinct diseases with overlapping presentations and separate etiologies. Evaporative dry eye, although frequently associated with aqueous deficiency, is also considered a separate entity. We propose viewing dry eye, both evaporative and insufficiency, as the natural sequelae of chronic blepharitis induced by biofilm. We suggest describing this one chronic disease as dry eye blepharitis syndrome (DEBS). The disease process begins when normal flora bacteria colonize the lid margin beginning shortly after birth. This colonization accompanies the development of a biofilm on the lid margin. As years pass, the biofilm matures, and the increased bacterial population initiates the production of inflammatory virulence factors, such as exotoxins, cytolytic toxins, and super-antigens, which persist on the lid margin for the rest of the patient's life. These virulence factors cause early follicular inflammation and later, meibomian gland dysfunction followed by aqueous insufficiency, and finally, after many decades, loss of the dense collagen in the tarsal plate. We proposed four stages of DEBS, which correlate with the clinical manifestations of folliculitis (anterior blepharitis), meibomitis (meibomian gland dysfunction), lacrimalitis (aqueous deficiency), and lid structure damage evidenced by increased lid laxity resulting in entropion, ectropion, and floppy eyelid syndrome.

Keywords: biofilm, blepharitis, demodex, dry eye disease, eyelids, meibomian glands, quorum-sensing gene activation, tear film

1. Introduction

Blepharitis was first described by ancient Egyptian physicians in the Ebers Papyrus, which prescribed potions such as "Cream with the Milk-of-a-Woman-who-has-borne-a-Son" [1, 2]. Despite centuries of study, little progress has been made in understanding or treating this disease. The long standing dogma of multifactorial, overlapping manifestations of blepharitis and dry eye have led to the use of inaccurate terminology that creates misunderstanding among both patients and providers [3, 4]. In order to develop our understanding of DEBS, we must first establish the correct use of the word blepharitis as suggested by the origin of the word (blepharon = lid, −itis = inflammation).

The next step in understanding dry eye disease and blepharitis as a single disease process is to identify the cause of eyelid inflammation. In 1954, Thygeson first recognized that blepharitis was associated with "abnormal Staphylococcus

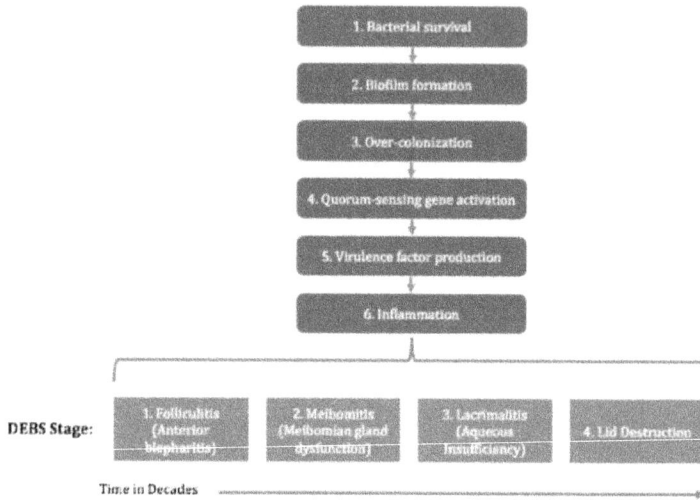

Figure 1.
Biofilm theory of dry eye disease: Schematic of six steps of bacterial biofilm development leading to the stages of DEBS.

colonization" of the eyelid margin [5]. Thygeson was describing the process by which our normal lid margin flora bacteria, primarily *Staphylococcus aureus* and *S. epidermidis*, gradually over-colonize the patient's lid margin, and over time, become pathogenic [6]. This is made possible by the bacterial biofilm, which allows the bacteria to thrive despite antimicrobials and the immune system [7]. Understanding biofilm progression links the shared underlying pathology between dry eye and blepharitis.

Biofilms are defined as groups of microbial cells enclosed in a matrix made primarily of polysaccharide material that are intimately associated with a surface. Antonie van Leeuwenhoek is credited for the first observations of biofilm, when he described the biofilm on teeth in 1684. However, further study of biofilms was limited until the development of the electron microscope in the mid-1900s. Furthermore, it was not until 1982 that the term "biofilm" was introduced, after Costerton's observation of a *S. aureus* biofilm on a cardiac pacemaker lead [8]. More recent studies have shown that cell-to-cell interactions ("quorum sensing") within the biofilm upregulate certain gene products. Further studies have implicated biofilm in many disease processes including periodontitis, endocarditis, chronic prostatitis, and medical device associated infections, as the one described by Costerton [8–10].

This chapter will explain the six steps by which our normal margin lid flora become pathogenic and cause eyelid inflammation. This inflammation, in turn, leads to the four stages of DEBS: folliculitis, meibomitis, lacrimalitis, and lid structure damage (**Figure 1**). This understanding will allow us to encompass dry eye disease, blepharitis, and meibomian gland dysfunction (MGD) in one disease process, namely, dry eye blepharitis syndrome (DEBS).

2. Biofilm

Bacteria were among the first forms of life on Earth and have survived billions of years in a myriad of different environments. While they are unicellular microorganisms, and can live in a free-floating form, the development of a biofilm provides them a strong, virtually impenetrable defense structure [8]. Furthermore, Absalon et al. and Pickering et al. suggest that free-floating bacteria are the minority in nature by describing the biofilm as "the prevailing microbial lifestyle" [11, 12].

The biofilm helps bacteria by acting as armor against host defense responses and desiccation. It enhances survival across species by allowing bacteria to produce virulence factors, concentrate nutrients, and communicate with other bacterial species [13]. Biofilms are involved in many infections and are present in almost any environment – they form plaque on the teeth and can lead to corrosion of metal pipes. They are involved in recurrent infections from medical devices – from sutures to prostheses. Although they can also be found as floating mats submerged in or on top of liquids, they are usually sticky and adhere easily to any surface [14]. For example, *S. epidermidis* and *S. aureus* produce a protein called "adhesin", which functions as a glue, ensuring a strong adhesion between the biofilm and its host surface [15]. Once adhered, they are hard to dislodge, allowing the bacteria to remain in a desirable environment.

Biofilms are likely to grow wherever there is moisture, nutrients, and a surface [16]. These are all present at the lid margin, which has the added benefit of its inherent warmth. It is well known that the lid margin is home to normal flora bacteria consisting of mainly coagulase-negative species such as *S. epidermidis* [6]. It is also well known that species of Staphylococcus, especially *S. epidermidis*, produce biofilms [17]. In addition, a recent study by Kivanç demonstrated that 32 out of 34 isolates cultured from eyes immediately after cataract surgery were positive for being biofilm-forming species [18]. Taking all this information into account, it should come as no surprise that biofilms easily develop on the lid margin.

Furthermore, to avoid irritating our eyes with soap when we wash our face, we instinctively keep our eyes tightly shut, lid margin against lid margin, effectively blocking access to an area that needs cleaning as much as or more than any other area of the body. Therefore, the biofilm accumulates microscopically year after year, layer upon layer, without any removal. Even if home scrubs are attempted, the adhesin "glue" can prevent biofilm elimination. As patients age, the biofilm continues to accrue, leading to each of the stages of DEBS over time. This process starts much earlier in contact lens wearers, since the contact lens is itself an inert foreign body, producing a very early biofilm that allows protection for bacteria. Biofilm formation on contact lens and contact lens cases has been well documented [19]. This also helps explain why dry eye disease is more common in contact lens wearers, 50% compared to 14% in controls [20].

The biofilm forms a multi-laminar substrate that provides more surface area for bacterial replication, which in turn leads to vast over-colonization of the surface. The over-colonization within the biofilm and increase in bacterial population density is what leads to quorum-sensing gene activation [21]. The discovery of quorum-sensing gene activation by Hastings in 1999, was a groundbreaking study that lead to increased understanding of bacterial virulence [22]. Hastings demonstrated that populations of bacteria can sense when their densities achieve a certain quorum, and once that number or density is reached, dormant genes are activated [23]. The bacteria signal to each other using chemical messengers called homoserine lactones (HSLs) as well as through electric currents produced by potassium ions [24]. When enough bacteria are in close proximity to each other, the signals from these the surrounding bacteria sum to indicate a quorum [25]. These newly activated genes produce a wide array of virulence factors, many of which are extremely inflammatory. The bacteria wait to produce these factors until they have the protective biofilm in place to shield from the host immune response [26]. The inflammation from the host response to these virulence factors is the real destructive force in inflammatory lid disease, causing low-grade, chronic inflammation, beginning on the lid surface, the structures of the lid margin such as lash follicles, meibomian glands and connective tissue, and eventually affecting the accessory lacrimal glands as it progresses.

S. epidermidis produces a small amount of a moderate cytolytic toxin, a phenol-soluble modulin, but *S. aureus* produces two groups of highly destructive and immunogenic exoproteins: exotoxins and enzymes [27–29]. Many exotoxins are super-antigens that signal T cells to secrete large amounts of cytokines, and thus, massive inflammation. Exotoxins are responsible for toxic shock syndrome, food poisoning and scalded skin syndrome (toxic shock syndrome toxin, staphylococcal enterotoxins A-E and G-I, and exfoliative toxins A and B respectively) [30, 31]. The enzymes produced consist of nucleases, proteases, lipases, hyaluronidase, and collagenase, all capable of destroying host tissue [32]. Cytolytic toxins, including hemolysins and leukocidins, further contribute to the inflammatory cascade by destroying or damaging cells [33].

These toxins and enzymes permeate the biofilm and its surroundings, creating the same massive inflammation that leads to acute, severe debilitating disease as in scalded skin syndrome, food poisoning, and even death, as in the case of toxic shock syndrome [34]. As the biofilm spreads, more areas reach the quorum needed to activate virulence factors. Thus, inflammation spreads from the lid margin, to within the lash follicles, meibomian glands, accessory lacrimal glands, possibly to the main lacrimal gland and eventually to nerve endings and even the connective tissue of the eyelid, which can affect the structural integrity of the eyelids [35]. Decades of this toxicity, and the resulting inflammation, leads to nonselective damage [36]. While the body manages to ward off some of the effects of this toxic environment until later in life, eventually no part of the lid is immune to this chronic, progressive inflammation [37].

3. The four stages of DEBS

As we have now established that inflammatory lid disease is due to the inflammatory response to virulence factors produced by a mature biofilm, we can proceed to understanding the various clinical manifestations of DEBS. The important factors to consider are lid anatomy, duration of biofilm presence and associated virulence factors along the lid margin. False descriptions such as anterior, posterior, staphylococcal or seborrheic do not accurately describe the stage of blepharitis, and merely serve as distractors. Instead, it is important to understand that inflammation is an inevitable consequence of virulence factor production, and it does not discriminate among structures of the lid. It simply takes some structures longer to be affected than others because of anatomy. Due to sticky proteins such as adhesin, as well as the biofilm's innate defense against antimicrobials and the immune system, the biofilm usually remains in place for most of the patient's life [38, 39]. This allows the inflammation to eventually affect all structures within the eyelid.

The biofilm is likely formed early in the patient's life, around the toddler stage. This early biofilm does not cause pathology in most cases because the densities of bacteria within the biofilm have not reached the quorum required to activate virulence factors. There are certainly exceptions, where children present with severe blepharitis [40]. These children likely have two particularly virulent strains of bacteria colonizing their eyelids simultaneously. The first is likely a hyper-virulent strain of *S. epidermidis*, which makes copious biofilm, and the second is a particularly virulent strain of *S. aureus*, whose quorum for gene activation is lower than normal [41] and whose toxins are more destructive. Further research into these children's lid flora would help clarify the variation in pathogenesis. Other factors such as rosacea and Demodex also remain to be investigated.

In the majority of the population, the biofilm must be present for decades before enough bacteria accumulate to reach a quorum [42]. As previously mentioned, biofilms form wherever there is a "combination of moisture, nutrients and a surface" [16]. Therefore, the lid margin, which provides all three of these requirements, is a logical starting point for the development of the biofilm. The lid margin includes the lash line and extends just past the openings of the meibomian glands [43]. Other areas of the ocular surface are better defended from the development of biofilm. Specifically, the mechanical sweeping and flushing of tears protects the palpebral and bulbar conjunctiva, while antibacterial lactoferrin and lysozyme protect the tear film [44–46]. Goblet cells provide further protection to the epithelial surfaces by secreting mucus [47].

Despite its antimicrobial protein content, the majority of the protection given by mucus is due to its mechanical characteristics. In the large intestine, there are two layers of mucus: the outer one houses gut bacteria, and the inner, impermeable layer prevents the underlying epithelial cells from bacterial invasion [48, 49]. While the small intestine lacks the inner layer, it still prevents bacterial exposure by creating a diffusion gradient with a rapid turnover that bacteria must overcome to access the epithelial cells [50]. Mucus trapping bacteria also prevent antigen presentation, which limits immune response. These functions may well help protect the conjunctiva as well – limiting environmental antigen presentation and forming an impenetrable barrier. In addition, the rapid turnover combined with the sweeping action of blinking creates an unstable surface to which a biofilm cannot adhere. Therefore, maintenance of a healthy population of goblet cells is essential to prevent biofilm buildup on the conjunctiva.

We know that the mucus is permeable to other molecules such as antibiotics, steroids, other medicated eye drops, therefore it is logical to assume that at least some of the exotoxins, enzymes and cytolytic toxins can reach the epithelia. Similarly, if virulence factors behave like the molecules in eye drops, it may be possible for them to slowly penetrate into the eye and damage structures within the eye; for example, the trabecular meshwork. Perhaps the meshwork simply becomes "sticky" due to subclinical inflammation and more easily traps protein, white cells or RBCs. This could occur through either subclinical inflammation or direct damage from cytolytic toxins and enzymes. If this is the case, it may in part explain why the incidence of glaucoma increases with age: a thicker biofilm releases more toxins which can damage lid margin structures and internal eye structures over time.

The manifestations of DEBS vary depending on the stage of the disease, which progresses exceedingly slowly. These differing presentations have led to confusion as to the presentation and progression of blepharitis and dry eye disease. This confusion stems from focusing on the presenting problem and not understanding what preceded it. For instance, if a patient has meibomian gland dysfunction, the diagnosis is made of evaporative dry eye disease, without further consideration of the lash follicles [51]. Similarly, if there is inadequate tear lake, the patient is diagnosed with aqueous insufficiency, ignoring the status of the meibomian glands [52, 53]. We hope to eliminate this confusion by dividing DEBS into four stages and by making a logical argument for the order of this progression based on eyelid anatomy and histology.

3.1 Stage 1: folliculitis (anterior blepharitis)

The first stage of DEBS involves the lash follicles. The potential space between the eyelash and the follicle surrounding it is easily invaded by the biofilm

(**Figure** 2). Once quorum densities are achieved and virulence factor production begins, the small lash bulb can become inflamed relatively quickly. Inflammation leads to edema, which can be clinically identified with the "volcano" sign – swollen follicular tissue around the base of the lash (**Figure 3**). The swollen tissue may also appear pale, possibly due transudate and/or capillary compression due to edema. The biofilm that adheres to the lash will be pulled along as the lash grows, result-ing in "collarettes" (**Figure 4**). These collarettes have also been called scurf, debris or lash dandruff. Because they originate from biofilm, they appear at different levels on the eyelash, depending on the lash's growth stage. Near the top of the lashes in **Figure 4**, it is possible to see collarettes just beginning to detach from the lid margin. This biofilm growth can also manifest as "cylindrical dandruff" [54]. Despite the term "dandruff," it is unlikely that sloughing layers of skin could form a cylinder around the eyelash. Thus, this term is most likely an inaccurate description of biofilm that accumulates around the lash base and sheathes the lash as it grows. Since the lash follicles are likely damaged through inflammation, the growth of the lash is slowed, which enables the biofilm accumulation to progress at the same rate as lash growth [55]. We have confirmed the presence of bacterial colonies in the scurf around lashes (**Figure 5**), and fluorescence microscopy was consistent with biofilm matrix around the lash [55].

A 2005 article by Gao et al. proposed that cylindrical dandruff was pathognomic for Demodex, which found that all their subjects who presented with cylindrical dandruff also had Demodex. While other studies had different findings, Gao et al. explained the discrepancy as "miscounting" by the other researchers [54]. However, even if the 100% incidence in this one study is completely accurate, correlation does not necessarily establish causation. A later article by Tsubota et al. found that "Demodex was detected in the cilia of 8 out of 10 (80%), and 22 cilia out of 30 (73%) with cylindrical dandruff" [56]. While these numbers certainly suggest an association, they do not imply causality. In fact, since Demodex were not detected in all of the lashes, it would suggest a lack of causality. Furthermore, Demodex does not extrude waste, instead storing it in its gut, which makes it unlikely that they secrete the dandruff [63]. It is much more likely that the eyelids accumulate an abundance of biofilm over time, which progresses along with eyelash growth,

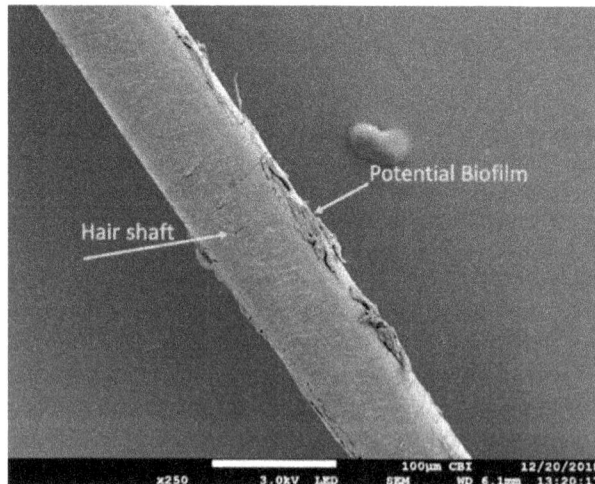

Figure 2.
Scanning electron microscopy of an eyelash hair shaft showing potential biofilm.

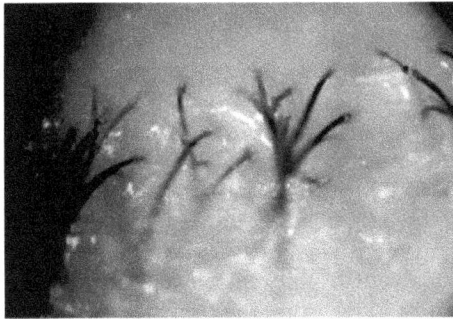

Figure 3.
The pallor around the lash follicles indicates the "volcano" sign associated with folliculitis.

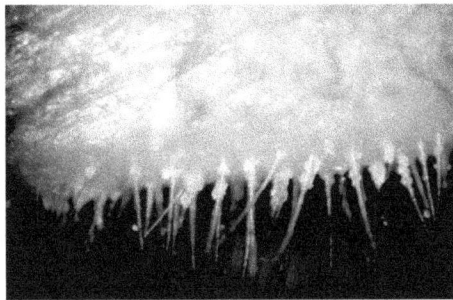

Figure 4.
Collarettes/cylindrical dandruff present on the lashes.

and that Demodex uses the polysaccharide biofilm as a rich source of nutrition. The cylindrical dandruff is likely a combination of Demodex carcasses and biofilm.

Collarettes, clumping, eye discharge, and sticky eyelids upon awakening are all evidence of bacterial biofilm along the lid margin. However, they are not required for diagnosis of blepharitis. In patients with late-stage disease, there may be significant lid inflammation without scurf. Though this may seem to be incongruous with blepharitis, the likely 40–50 years of inflammation at this stage have so badly damaged the eyelash bulb that the lashes are either barely growing or not growing at all. Therefore, there is no scurf, because there has been no/minimal lash growth to pull it away from the lid margin. Therefore, a paucity of lashes, in association with swollen lash follicles, as shown in **Figure 3**, can also indicate DEBS. In addition, these late-stage patients typically have exceedingly dry lid margins, which inhibit further biofilm production. In other words, bacteria can eventually become their own worst enemy by destroying the very moisture that is required for biofilm production.

3.2 Stage 2: meibomitis (MGD)

The next stage of DEBS involves the spread of inflammation from the lash follicles to the meibomian glands. These glands are relatively more protected than the follicles due to their narrow ductules and the constant flow of meibum out of the gland. These characteristics ensure that meibomian involvement occurs after follicular involvement. Meibomian glands are also 5–10 times larger than lash follicles, which means that inflammation takes longer to significantly hinder the working of the gland than the follicle [57]. The amount of time between Stage 1 and Stage 2 depends on the virulence and biofilm production characteristics of the patient's particular bacterial profile, but we estimate approximately 10–15 years between them.

Obvious vs. nonobvious MGD is a recent topic of discussion and can also be explained through understanding the biofilm. Obvious MGD manifests with inspissation and capping (domes over gland openings) that can be observed on exam (**Figure 6**). On the other hand, nonobvious MGD does not have these manifestations. Nonobvious MGD can be thought of as the biofilm forming layers within the gland and starting the inflammatory process [58]. As the biofilm accumulates within the gland and mixes with meibum, it eventually blocks the narrow ductule, thereby causing obstruction. This thickened mixture of biofilm and meibum takes on a "toothpaste" quality and may alter the consistency of the lipid profile of the meibum, either through the presence of abnormal lipids or decreased overall lipid secretion [59]. The mixture of meibum with biofilm has an increased melting point, which leads to thickening and obstruction. These secretions may not be expressed because the meibomian glands are large and the biofilm may not have affected a significant enough portion of them yet, therefore leading to nonobvious MGD. Once the gland is full of the thick meibum and biofilm mixture, the secretions will have

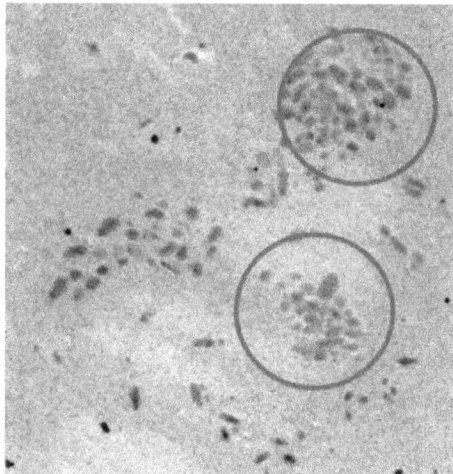

Figure 5.
Transmission electron microscopy of cylindrical dandruff showing bacterial colonies (blue circles), which suggests that the dandruff is likely biofilm.

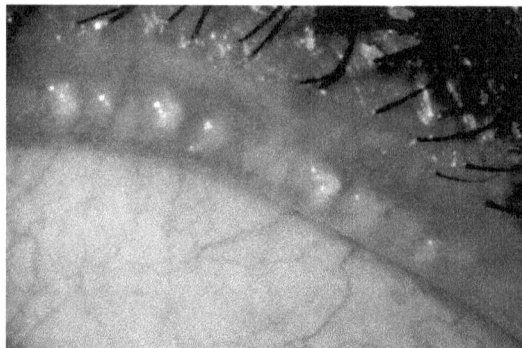

Figure 6.
Evidence of meibomian gland dysfunction showing inspissation and capping.

nowhere further to accumulate within the gland and will attempt to move up and out of the ductule. However, the original biofilm traps these secretions forming small whitish domes similar in color to what is observed within an early non-obvious occluded ductule. Expression of the glands may release copious amounts of sludge or inspissated secretions. While the composition of the peaks or caps has never been effectively studied, it is not difficult to imagine that they are composed of accumulated "altered" meibum mixed with biofilm covered by a more "pure" biofilm [60]. Therefore, the filling of the gland past its capacity is what triggers the appearance of the "domes" in obvious MGD, but it is the thickened biofilm mixture which has reached quorum-sensing that begins the early, and later obvious, signs of overt inflammation along the posterior lid margin [61]. Hence, the difference between obvious and nonobvious MGD is simply one of degree.

3.3 Stage 3: lacrimalitis (aqueous deficiency)

Stage 3 DEBS involvement of the accessory lacrimal glands of Wolfring and Krause, and probably the main lacrimal gland, leads to aqueous deficiency. There are approximately 30 lacrimal glands of Krause and about 5 glands of Wolfring on each eye. They are responsible for baseline aqueous production [62, 63]. The ducts of these glands empty along the inside lid, up near the fornices. The distance from the lid margin biofilm, the narrow ducts, and the constant flushing activity of tear production all serve to protect these glands from activity along the lid margin. However, the biofilm can spread from the lid margin by being shed into the tear film, and decades of shedding eventually leads to some biofilm infiltrating the glands of Krause and Wolfring. Alternatively, it is quite possible that a layer of biofilm, kept attenuated due to constant flushing and lid/eye movement, nevertheless eventually reaches these glands by direct extension. Because of their innately protective distance from the lid margin, these glands are the last group to become infiltrated by biofilm, and therefore, the last to succumb to the effects of inflammatory damage from biofilm virulence factors. This is supported by looking at clinical manifestations of patients with many of the symptoms of dry eye – burning, irritation, and difficulty seeing – in conjunction with excessive tearing. While exam may lead to diagnosis of evaporative dry eye with a deficient lipid layer, patients may not understand how they could have dry yet watery eyes. These patients have deficient lipid production but intact aqueous production, indicating diseased meibomian glands but still healthy accessory glands of Krause and Wolfring. On the other hand, unless there is an autoimmune disorder, it is virtually impossible to see an aqueous-deficient patient without MGD (**Figure 7**). This finding supports the conclusion that aqueous deficiency presents after evaporative dry eye due to the accessory lacrimal glands being affected after the meibomian glands.

By the time we have Stage 3 DEBS, the follicles have been subjected to chronic inflammation for many decades and are sometimes so badly damaged that lash growth is arrested, and hence, there may be little-to-no biofilm noted among the eyelashes. Lashes fall out and may not regrow or regrow very slowly. Looking closely, one will typically find significant swelling around the base of the lash along with pallor as in Stage 1.

3.4 Stage 4: lid destruction

Stage 4 DEBS is marked by the breakdown of the structural integrity of the eyelid. Lid laxity, entropion, ectropion, and floppy eyelid syndrome are often manifestations of end-stage chronic inflammatory lid disease [64]. The inflammation associated with the formation of the biofilm eventually affects connective tissue,

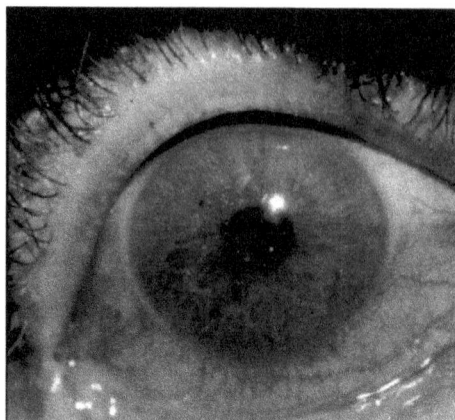

Figure 7.
Eye showing both aqueous deficiency (positive staining with rose Bengal) and meibomian gland dysfunction (pouting of glands).

muscle, and nerve endings within the lid margin, which become damaged and lose their functionality [65]. Because of the loss of the nerve endings, these patients are often asymptomatic. Also, as mentioned prior, since bacteria need moisture to grow and produce biofilms, years of dry eye may degrade their once-ideal environment to the point where they cannot sustain large colonies of bacteria, these patients often present with little to no biofilm. By this point, however, the damage to the lid and the tear glands is already done and may be irreversible.

3.5 Management

The armor provided by the polysaccharide matrix of the biofilm explains why many novel treatments proposed in the past 100 years have failed. The only treatment for chronic blepharitis universally agreed upon is lid hygiene [66]. Historically we have preferred simple salt water soaks [67]. Recently, microblepharoexfoliation (MBE) has become available [68]. This additional form of lid hygiene provides a thorough mechanical biofilm removal of the lid margin, which may have a profound impact on patient's symptoms, quality of tears, and quality of life. Therefore, we propose performing MBE of patients' lids, with electric rotary sponge cleaning, in an effort to remove the biofilm and prevent and/or slow down the progression of DEBS (**Figure 8**).

Besides the treatment of DEBS, MBE may have other potential roles in ophthalmology. It is known that endophthalmitis is most commonly associated with the presence of biofilm-forming bacteria in the patients' lid margin. The aforementioned Kivanç study demonstrated that these biofilm formers are present and can survive a Betadine wash [18]. By performing a thorough MBE of the patient's lids, we may be able to reduce the incidence of post-cataract infection. In addition, by removing the biofilm from the lid margin and meibomian glands, we should expect a better tear film and therefore more accurate pre-operative screening and, more importantly, better post-op vision. Similarly, patients undergoing refractive surgery, such as laser in situ keratomileusis, photorefractive keratectomy, and phototherapeutic keratectomy, and contact lens wearers will probably also benefit from an electromechanical debridement of their lid margin. All of these patients may benefit from the reduction or elimination of the progression of the lid biofilm with yearly electromechanical debridement.

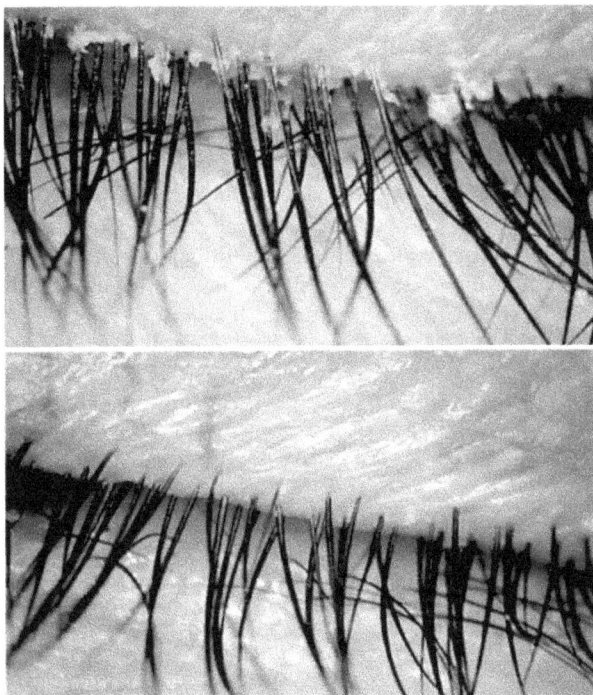

Figure 8.
Upper lid lash margin showing presence of cylindrical dandruff and "scurf". Top: Before MBE; Bottom: After MBE (Courtesy of BlephEx, Inc.).

4. Conclusions

Understanding DEBS as a singular disease process that presents in stages, over decades, throughout a person's lifetime allows us to successfully explain all clinical scenarios we encounter. DEBS explains the overlap of the so-called anterior blepharitis with posterior blepharitis, why we do not see isolated cases of aqueous deficiency and why the disease worsens with age. It also shows why some patients may become asymptomatic and why we sometimes do not see biofilm within the lash line despite severe lid disease findings. Finally, DEBS also describes chronic changes to the structural integrity of the eyelids, including lash loss.

Dentists have done a masterful job in educating patients as to the importance of routine oral hygiene. "Plaque" has become a household term for dental biofilm. While in the past years of biofilm-related inflammation caused elderly patients to require dentures, patient education is helping full dentures become obsolete. In 2006, a CDC report claimed "the baby boomer generation will be the first where the majority will maintain their natural teeth over their entire lifetime" [69].

We too can improve patient outcomes by preventing damage to the critically important meibomian glands and other eyelid structures, rather than reacting to the damage once it is already done. To prevent DEBS, we need to make routine lid hygiene akin to "brushing your teeth" and electromechanical debridement as commonplace as routine dental cleaning. This is now possible, but it must start with a new understanding of DEBS, and an active role by the ophthalmologist stressing lid hygiene and advocating for regular MBE procedures on all patients, the sooner the better, particularly on those at higher risk.

Acknowledgements

We would like to thank Dr. Donna B. Stolz, Dr. Michael B. Choi, Dr. Michael Hadjiargyrou and Nicole Radova, B.S. for their contributions to this chapter.

Conflict of interest

James M Rynerson is the President and CEO of BlephEx, LLC and Henry D Perry is the senior founding partner of Ophthalmic Consultants of Long Island. The authors report no other conflicts of interest in this work.

Appendices and nomenclature

Biofilm	Groups of microbial cells enclosed in a matrix of primarily polysaccharide material that are intimately associated with a surface
Blepharitis	Inflammation of the eyelid
Cylindrical dandruff	Sleeve of material that forms around the eyelash, likely due to biofilm accumulation combined with eyelash growth
DEBS	Dry Eye Blepharitis Syndrome; a proposed unifying diagnosis that links both dry eye and blepharitis as stages of inflammation caused by progression of biofilm
Goblet cells	Specialized epithelial cells that secrete mucus, helping maintain the barrier against pathogens
Microblepharoexfoliation (MBE)	Lid margin cleaning, with electric rotary sponge, in an effort to remove accumulated biofilm
Virulence factors	Factors released by bacteria that cause inflammation, including exotoxins, enzymes, super-antigens and cytolytic toxins
Volcano sign	Swollen, follicular tissue around the base of the lash

Biofilm Theory for Lid Margin and Dry Eye Disease
DOI: http://dx.doi.org/10.5772/intechopen.89969

Author details

Maria Vincent[1], Jose Quintero[2], Henry D. Perry[1,2*] and James M. Rynerson[3]

1 Donald and Barbara Zucker School of Medicine at Hofstra/Northwell, New York, USA

2 Ophthalmic Consultants of Long Island, New York, USA

3 BlephEx LLC, Kentucky, USA

*Address all correspondence to: hankcornea@gmail.com

IntechOpen

References

[1] Bryan CP. Ancient Egyptian Medicine: The Papyrus Ebers. London: Ares; 1930. p. 95

[2] Andersen SR. The eye and its diseases in ancient Egypt. Acta Ophthalmologica Scandinavica. 1997;75:338-344

[3] Dougherty JM, McCulley JP. Analysis of the free fatty acid component of meibomian secretions in chronic blepharitis. Investigative Ophthalmology & Visual Science. 1986;27(1):52-56

[4] Foulks GN. The correlation between the tear film lipid layer and dry eye disease. Survey of Ophthalmology. 2007;52(4):369-374. DOI: 10.1016/j.survophthal.2007.04.009

[5] Thygeson P, Vaughan DG Jr. Seborrheic blepharitis. Transactions of the American Ophthalmological Society. 1954;52:173-188

[6] Dougherty JM, McCulley JP. Comparative bacteriology of chronic blepharitis. The British Journal of Ophthalmology. 1984;68(8):524-528. DOI: 10.1136/bjo.68.8.524

[7] Brothers KM, Nau AC, Romanowski EG, Shanks RM. Dexamethasone diffusion across contact lenses is inhibited by *Staphylococcus epidermidis* biofilms *in vitro*. Cornea. 2014;33(10):1083-1087. DOI: 10.1097/ICO.0000000000000196

[8] Del Pozo JL. Biofilm-related disease. Expert Review of Anti-Infective Therapy. 2018;16(1):51-65. DOI: 10.1080/14787210.2018.1417036

[9] Donlan RM. Biofilms: Microbial life on surfaces. Emerging Infectious Diseases. 2002;8(9):881-890. DOI: 10.3201/eid0809.020063

[10] Donlan RM. Biofilms and device-associated infections. Emerging

Infectious Diseases. 2001;7(2):277-281. DOI: 10.3201/eid0702.010226

[11] Absalon C, Van Dellen K, Watnick P. A communal bacterial adhesin anchors biofilm and bystander cells to surfaces. PLoS Pathogens. 2011;7(8):e1002210. DOI: 10.1371/journal.ppat.1002210

[12] Pickering BS, Smith DR, Watnick PJ. Glucose-specific enzyme IIA has unique binding partners in the *Vibrio cholerae* biofilm. MBio. 2012;3(6):e00228-e00212. DOI: 10.1128/mBio.00228-12

[13] Teles R, Teles F, Frias-Lopez F, Paster B, Haffajee A. Lessons learned and unlearned in periodontal microbiology. Periodontology 2000. 2013;2000, 62(1):95-162. DOI: 10.1111/prd.12010

[14] Costerton JW, Cheng KJ, Geesey GG, Ladd TI, Nickel JC, Dasgupta M, et al. Bacterial biofilms in nature and disease. Annual Review of Microbiology. 1987;41:435-464. DOI: 10.1146/annurev.mi.41.100187.002251

[15] Edwards AM, Bowden MG, Brown EL, Laabei M, Masey RC. *Staphylococcus aureus* extracellular adherence protein triggers TNFα release, promoting attachment to endothelial cells via protein A. PLoS One. 2012;7(8):e43046. DOI: 10.1371/journal.pone.0043046

[16] Weiser J, Henke HA, Hector N, et al. Sub-inhibitorytigecyclineconcentrations induce extracellular matrix binding protein Embp dependent Staphylococcus epidermidis biofilm formation and immune evasion. International Journal of Medical Microbiology. 2016;306(6):471-478. DOI: 10.1016/j.ijmm.2016.05.015

[17] Paharik AE, Horswill AR. The staphylococcal biofilm: Adhesins,

regulation, and host response. Microbiology Spectrum. 2016;**4**(2):22-215. DOI: 10.1128/microbiolspec. VMBF-0022-2015

[18] Kıvanç SA, Kıvanç M, Bayramlar H. Microbiology of corneal wounds after cataract surgery: Biofilm formation and antibiotic resistance patterns. Journal of Wound Care. 2016;**25**(1):12, 14-12, 19. DOI: 10.12968/jowc.2016.25.1.12, 10.1128/JB.182.10.2675-2679.2000

[19] Artini M, Cellini A, Scoarughi GL, et al. Evaluation of contact lens multipurpose solutions on bacterial biofilm development. Eye & Contact Lens. 2015;**41**(3):177-182. DOI: 10.1097/ ICL.0000000000000105

[20] Khaireddin R, Hueber A. Eyelid hygiene for contact lens wearers with blepharitis. Comparative investigation of treatment with baby shampoo versus phospholipid solution. Der Ophthalmologe. 2013;**110**(2):146-153. German. DOI: 10.1007/ s00347-012-2725-6

[21] Wolf D, Rippa V, Mobarec JC, et al. The quorum-sensing regulator ComA from Bacillus subtilis activates transcription using topologically distinct DNA motifs. Nucleic Acids Research. 2016;**44**(5):2160-2172. DOI: 10.1093/nar/gkv1242

[22] Davis TH. Profile of J woodland Hastings. Proceedings of the National Academy of Sciences of the United States of America. 2007;**104**(3):693-695. DOI: 10.1073/pnas.0610519104

[23] Hastings JW, Greenberg EP. Quorum sensing: The explanation of a curious phenomenon reveals a common characteristic of bacteria. Journal of Bacteriology. 1999;**181**(9):2667-2668

[24] Mireille Ayé A, Bonnin-Jusserand M, Brian-Jaisson F, et al. Modulation of violacein production and phenotypes associated with

biofilm by exogenous quorum sensing N-acylhomoserine lactones in the marine bacterium. Pseudoalteromonas ulvae TC14. Microbiology. 2015;**161**(10):2039-2051. DOI: 10.1099/ mic.0.000147

[25] Zhang C, Zhu S, Jatt AN, Zeng M. Characterization of N-acyl homoserine lactones (AHLs) producing bacteria isolated from vacuum-packaged refrigerated turbot (Scophthalmus maximus) and possible influence of exogenous AHLs on bacterial phenotype. The Journal of General and Applied Microbiology. 2016;**62**(2):60-67. DOI: 10.2323/jgam.62.60

[26] Knecht LD, O'Connor G, Mittal R, et al. Serotonin activates bacterial quorum sensing and enhances the virulence of Pseudomonas aeruginosa in the host. eBioMedicine. 2016;**9**:161-169. DOI: 10.1016/j. ebiom.2016.05.037

[27] Cheung GY, Joo HS, Chatterjee SS, Otto M. Phenol-soluble modulins – Critical determinants of staphylococcal virulence. FEMS Microbiology Reviews. 2014;**38**(4):698-719. DOI: 10.1111/1574-6976.12057

[28] Prince LR, Graham KJ, Connolly J, et al. Staphylococcus aureus induces eosinophil cell death mediated by α-hemolysin. PLoS One. 2012;**7**(2):e31506. DOI: 10.1371/journal. pone.0031506

[29] Stroh P, Günther F, Meyle E, Prior B, Wagner C, Hänsch GM. Host defence against Staphylococcus aureus biofilms by polymorphonuclear neutrophils: Oxygen radical production but not phagocytosis depends on opsonisation with immunoglobulin G. Immunobiology. 2011;**216**(3):351-357. DOI: 10.1016/j.imbio.2010.07.009

[30] Liew YK, Awang Hamat R, van Belkum A, Chong PP, Neela V. Comparative exoproteomics and

host inflammatory response in Staphylococcus aureus skin and soft tissue infections, bacteremia, and subclinical colonization. Clinical and Vaccine Immunology. 2015;**22**(5):593-603. DOI: 10.1128/CVI.00493-14

[31] Holmes A, Ganner M, McGuane S, Pitt TL, Cookson BD, Kearns AM. Staphylococcus aureus isolates carrying Panton-valentine leucocidin genes in England and Wales: Frequency, characterization, and association with clinical disease. Journal of Clinical Microbiology. 2005;**43**(5):2384-2390. DOI: 10.1128/JCM.43.5.2384-2390.2005

[32] Maloney WJ, Smith RL, Castro F, Schurman DJ. Fibroblast response to metallic debris in vitro. Enzyme induction cell proliferation, and toxicity. The Journal of Bone and Joint Surgery. American Volume. 1993;**75**(6):835-844. DOI: 10.2106/00004623-199306000-00005

[33] Dinges MM, Orwin PM, Schlievert PM. Exotoxins of Staphylococcus aureus. Clinical Microbiology Reviews. 2000;**13**(1):16-34. DOI: 10.1128/cmr.13.1.16-34.2000

[34] Krakauer T. Update on staphylococcal superantigen-induced signaling pathways and therapeutic interventions. Toxins (Basel). 2013;**5**(9):1629-1654. DOI: 10.3390/toxins5091629

[35] Baudouin CJ. Un nouveau schéma pour mieux comprendre les maladies de la surface oculaire. [a new approach for better comprehension of diseases of the ocular surface]. Journal Français d'Ophtalmologie. 2007;**30**(3):239-246. French. DOI: JFO-03-2007-30-3-0181-5512-101019-200700462

[36] Brüning T, Bartsch R, Bolt HM, et al. Sensory irritation as a basis for setting occupational exposure limits. Archives of Toxicology.

2014;**88**(10):1855-1879. DOI: 10.1007/s00204-014-1346-z

[37] Pflugfelder SC, Stern ME. Symposium participants Immunoregulation on the ocular surface: 2nd Cullen symposium. The Ocular Surface. 2009;**7**(2):67-77. DOI: 10.1016/S1542-0124(12)70297-5

[38] Suzuki T, Kawamura Y, Uno T, Ohashi Y, Ezaki T. Prevalence of Staphylococcus epidermidis strains with biofilm-forming ability in isolates from conjunctiva and facial skin. American Journal of Ophthalmology. 2005;**140**(5):844-850. DOI: 10.1016/j.ajo.2005.05.050

[39] Miyanaga Y. A new perspective in ocular infection and the role of antibiotics. Ophthalmologica. 1997;**211**(Suppl 1):9-14. DOI: 10.1159/000310879

[40] Cetinkaya A, Akova YA. Pediatric ocular acne rosacea: Long-term treatment with systemic antibiotics. American Journal of Ophthalmology. 2006;**142**(5):816-821. DOI: 10.1016/j.ajo.2006.06.047

[41] Nazir SA, Murphy S, Siatkowski RM, Chodosh J, Siatkowski RL. Ocular rosacea in childhood. American Journal of Ophthalmology. 2004;**137**(1):138-144. DOI: 10.1016/S0002-9394(03)00890-0

[42] Huse HK, Kwon T, Zlosnik JE, Speert DP, Marcotte EM, Whiteley M. Pseudomonas aeruginosa enhances production of a non-alginate exopolysaccharide during long-term colonization of the cystic fibrosis lung. PLoS One. 2013;**8**(12):e82621. DOI: 10.1371/journal.pone.0082621

[43] Pflugfelder SC, Karpecki PM, Perez VL. Treatment of blepharitis: Recent clinical trials. The Ocular Surface. 2014;**12**(4):273-284. DOI: 10.1016/j.jtos.2014.05.005

[44] Pult H, Riede-Pult BH, Murphy PJ. A new perspective on spontaneous blinks. Ophthalmology. 2013;**120**(5):1086-1091. DOI: 10.1016/j.ophtha.2012.11.010

[45] Albar AH, Almehdar HA, Uversky VN, Redwan EM. Structural heterogeneity and multifunctionality of lactoferrin. Current Protein & Peptide Science. 2014;**15**(8):778-797. DOI: 10.1152/ajpcell.1991.260.2.C183

[46] Tiffany JM. The normal tear film. Developments in Ophthalmology. 2008;**41**:1-20. DOI: 10.1159/000131066

[47] Dartt DA, Masli S. Conjunctival epithelial and goblet cell function in chronic inflammation and ocular allergic inflammation. Current Opinion in Allergy and Clinical Immunology. 2014;**14**(5):464-470. DOI: 10.1097/ACI.0000000000000098

[48] Galley JD, Yu Z, Kumar P, Dowd SE, Lyte M, Bailey MT. The structures of the colonic mucosa-associated and luminal microbial communities are distinct and differentially affected by a prolonged murine stressor. Gut Microbes. 2014;**5**(6):748-760. DOI: 10.4161/19490976.2014.972241

[49] Johansson ME. Mucus layers in inflammatory bowel disease. Inflammatory Bowel Diseases. 2014;**20**(11):2124-2131. DOI: 10.1097/MIB.0000000000000117

[50] Johansson ME, Jakobsson HE, Holmén-Larsson J, et al. Normalization of host intestinal mucus layers requires long-term microbial colonization. Cell Host & Microbe. 2015;**18**(5):582-592. DOI: 10.1016/j.chom.2015.10.007

[51] Uchiyama E, Aronowicz JD, Butovich IA, McCulley JP. Pattern of vital staining and its correlation with aqueous tear deficiency and meibomian gland dropout. Eye & Contact Lens. 2007;**33**(4):177-179. DOI: 10.1097/01.icl.0000253054.10349.2f

[52] Messmer EM. The pathophysiology, diagnosis, and treatment of dry eye disease. Deutsches Ärzteblatt International. 2015;**112**(5):71-81. DOI: 10.3238/arztebl.2015.0071

[53] Yeotikar NS, Zhu H, Markoulli M, Nichols KK, Naduvilath T, Papas EB. Functional and morphologic changes of meibomian glands in an asymptomatic adult population. Investigative Ophthalmology & Visual Science. 2016;**57**(10):3996-4007. DOI: 10.1167/iovs.15-18467

[54] Gao YY, Di Pascuale MA, Li W, et al. High prevalence of Demodex in eyelashes with cylindrical dandruff. Investigative Ophthalmology & Visual Science. 2005;**46**(9):3089-3094. DOI: 10.1167/iovs.05-0275

[55] Choi MB, Stolz DB, Chu R, Grillo L, Donnenfeld ED, Perry HD. Histopathologic evaluation of pipe stemming cylindrical dandruff and debris on eyelash base in patients with blepharitis. In: Poster Presented at Association for Research in Vision and Ophthalmology 2019 Annual Meeting: 2019 Apr 28–May 02, Vancouver BC.

[56] Kawakita T, Kawashima M, Ibrahim O, Murato D, Tsubota K. Demodex-related marginal blepharitis in Japan. Nippon Ganka Gakkai Zasshi. 2010;**114**(12):1025-1029. Japanese

[57] Elder MJ. Anatomy and physiology of eyelash follicles: Relevance to lash ablation procedures. Ophthalmic Plastic and Reconstructive Surgery. 1997;**13**(1):21-25

[58] Blackie CA, Korb DR, Knop E, Bedi R, Knop N, Holland EJ. Nonobvious obstructive meibomian gland dysfunction. Cornea. 2010;**29**(12):1333-1345. DOI: 10.1097/ICO.0b013e3181d4f366

[59] Gao Y, Zhuang M, Fan C, Ye K, Hu J, Hong Y. Abnormal property of meibomian secretion and dry eye syndrome. Yan Ke Xue Bao. 2007;**23**(2):121-125. Chinese

[60] Uzunosmanoglu E, Mocan MC, Kocabeyoglu S, Karakaya J, Irkec M. Meibomian gland dysfunction in patients receiving long-term glaucoma medications. Cornea. 2016;**35**(8):1112-1116. DOI: 10.1097/ICO.0000000000000838

[61] Knop I, Korb DR, Blackie CA, Knop N. The lid margin is an underestimated structure for preservation of ocular surface health and development of dry eye disease. Developments in Ophthalmology. 2010;**45**:108-122. DOI: 10.1159/000315024

[62] Conrady CD, Joos ZP, Patel BC. Review: The lacrimal gland and its role in dry eye. Journal of Ophthalmology. 2016;**2016**:7542929. DOI: 10.1155/2016/7542929

[63] Stevenson W, Pugazhendhi S, Wang M. Is the main lacrimal gland indispensable? Contributions of the corneal and conjunctival epithelia. Survey of Ophthalmology. 2016;**61**(5):616-627. DOI: 10.1155/2016/7542929

[64] Baudouin C, Messmer EM, Aragona P, et al. Revisiting the vicious circle of dry eye disease: A focus on the pathophysiology of meibomian gland dysfunction. The British Journal of Ophthalmology. 2016;**100**(3):300-306. DOI: 10.1136/bjophthalmol-2015-307415

[65] Baudouin C. Ocular surface and external filtration surgery: Mutual relationships. Developments in Ophthalmology. 2012;**50**:64-78. DOI: 10.1159/000334791

[66] Lindlsey K, Matsumara S, Hatef E, Akpek EK. Interventions for chronic blepharitis. Cochrane Database of Systematic Reviews. 2012;**5**:CD005556. DOI: 10.1002/14651858.CD005556.pub2

[67] Romero JM, Biser SA, Perry HD, et al. Conservative treatment of meibomian gland dysfunction. Eye & Contact Lens. 2004;**30**(1):14-19. DOI: 10.1097/01.ICL.0000095229.01957.89

[68] Murphy O, O'Dwyer V, Lloyd-McKernan A. The efficacy of tea tree face wash, 1, 2-Octanediol and microblepharoexfoliation in treating Demodex folliculorum blepharitis. Contact Lens & Anterior Eye. 2018;**41**(1):77-82. DOI: 10.1016/j.clae.2017.10.012

[69] Miller R. The Slow Fade of False Teeth [Internet]. 2010. Available from: https://www.newstimes.com/news/article/The-slow-fade-of-false-teeth-599801.php [Accessed: 26 August 2019]

Chapter 3

Hyperosmolarity of the Tear Film in the Dry Eye

Alejandro Aguilar and Alejandro Berra

Abstract

The dry eye is a complex multifactor illness of the tear film and of the ocular surface characterized by symptoms of discomfort, vision alterations, and instability of the pre-corneal tear film which may bring about potential damage on the ocular surface. Instability of the film will produce increasing osmolarity of the tear film which will trigger epithelium osmotic lesions and inflammation. As these changes take place on the ocular surface, neurophysiologic mechanisms of homeostasis will be altered which will complicate the process even further with the cropping of vicious physiopathologic circuits.

Keywords: dry eye, tear film, hyperosmolarity, inflammation, physiopathologic circuits

1. Introduction

The ocular surface is a delicate portion of the eye's anatomy, where its constituent components maintain a close relationship in order to keep the region's homeostasis, which undoubtedly establishes the presence of a real anatomo-functional unit [1] in which the tear film must uphold the unimpaired health of epithelia of the conjunctiva and cornea and at the same time contribute to the normal physiology of the stroma.

In order that the tear film may carry out this function efficiently, its three layers must be complete and in constant equilibrium. The film's three layers have a close relationship, to such an extent, that any alteration in one of them (composition, secretory, etc.) may drastically impinge on the normal equilibrium of all, thus bringing about the partial or total alteration of the tear film and consequently alteration of the tear film and consequently altering epithelia.

2. Physiology

The dry eye is a pathologic multifactor process of the ocular surface due to a deficiency in quantity and/or quality of the pre-corneal tear film, which in turn makes it unable to keep healthy the epithelia of the cornea and the conjunctiva. This produces epithelial metaplasia of the squamous type and epithelial damage [2].

Even though this flaw may be due to different situations, increase of evaporation, deficiency in its production, and alteration in composition, in all cases the physiopathologic sequence is the increase of the film's osmolarity [3] which appears within the first 24 h of the onset of the process.

The decrease in the production of tears and/or qualitative changes in composition and also the evaporation of the film promote the phenomenon of hyperosmolarity. The evaporation of a smaller volume for a same surface increases osmolarity during the first 24 h from the onset of volumetric decrease [4].

Hyperosmolarity [5] causes epithelial injury in a direct manner as it produces cellular desquamation, complete disappearance of layers of superficial epithelial cells, decreasing of cytoplasmic density, and accumulation of rows of mucus product of goblet cells osmotically altered. This phenomenon is generally evident between 15 and 30 days from the osmolar change of the tear film.

According to Holly and Lamberts [6], the formation of the pre-corneal tear film is essentially a phenomenon of "wettability." The epithelium of the cornea and conjunctiva must be completely humidified by the aqueous layer of the film. For a complete wettability, the conditions of the ocular surface need that the surface tension of the aqueous layer in the interphase with the epithelium be lower than the surface tension of the epithelium exposed to the medium.

Mucopolysaccharides of the mucin layer are principally responsible in keeping a stable surface tension. Mucus accumulation and destruction of goblet cells due to an increase of the film's osmolarity brings about an increase in the surface tension, and therefore the wettability of the epithelium is inhibited.

In 1993 I advanced a hypothesis [7] based on the phenomenon of osmosis. The principle of osmosis is characterized by the presence of a solvent flow through a semipermeable membrane, which comes about when the concentration of the solution increases on one of the sides of the membrane. This aqueous movement tends to equalize concentrations on both sides [8]. When this occurs the osmotic phenomenon stops.

The corneal-conjunctival epithelium and the mucin layer of the tear film constitute a perfect biological semipermeable membrane and therefore act as such. When the osmolarity of the aqueous layer increases, the osmotic phenomenon begins producing a solvent flow from the epithelia and mucin layer towards the aqueous layer. This flow, nourished by the osmotic pressure, generates an important force that separates the aqueous layer impeding wettability.

At the same time, dehydration produced in the mucin layer will bring about destruction of mucus which raises higher surface tension, boosting osmolar disequilibrium.

At this point *sicca* lesion has taken place; it is exacerbated with cellular dehydration of the cellular layers of the epithelium generated in the aforementioned process and enters into a physiopathologic vicious circle.

On the other hand, taking into account the presence of the aqueous gradient through the protein water canals present in the stroma and with direction towards the aqueous humor, we shall observe that a new physical force of opposite direction (osmotic force) may modify this movement. This directional change of fluids produced by hyperosmolarity and by the mechanisms it produces may bring about dehydration of sulfated proteoglycans (GAGS) which occupy the spaces among collagen fibers of the stroma [9, 10]. When these glycoproteic structures dehydrate, the correct hydric balance of the stroma will be affected, which will incide in the normal maintenance of transparency of the cornea. Concurrently, alteration of the stroma will produce a loss in the number of goblet cells, with ensuing mucin and tensional alteration formerly described [11].

In this way, hyperosmolarity triggers a series of physiopathologic phenomena with evident feedback effects among them, which in both directions boost each other.

It is germane to this analysis that increase of osmolarity of the tear film in the dry eye, as a condition of stress on the ocular surface, triggers the inflammatory process and immunologic phenomena as the presence of autoantigens that boost the inflammatory process.

Studies on inflammatory markers such as NF-Kβ that migrates from the nucleus to the cytoplasm in the inflammatory process are directly related with the phenomenon of hyperosmolarity of the tear film. Nuclear translocation of NF-Kβ is directly proportional to the increase of osmolarity of the tear film.

Berra and Berra [12] compared the nuclear NF-Kβ translocation in healthy persons, in postmenopausal women, and in patients with Sjögren's syndrome, and they related them with osmolarity of the tear film and with impression cytology of these patients.

Healthy persons with normal values of osmolarity (300 mOsm/L ± 10) did not show presence of marker NF-Kβ, nor did they show metaplastic changes in the conjunctiva (normal cytology grade 0, according to Nelson's Classification) [13]. Postmenopausal women carriers of a moderate dry eye showed a moderate increase of osmolarity of the tear film (300–400 mOsm/L), moderate presence of factor NF-Kβ, and cellular metaplastic alterations grades I–II. On the contrary, patients with a severe dry eye, group with Sjögren's syndrome, showed high values of osmolarity of the film (>400 mOsm/L), a great expression of nuclear translocation of factor NF-Kβ, and severe squamous metaplasia (grades II–III).

Khanal et al. [14] compared values of the tear film's osmolarity in healthy persons with patients with dry eye, providing hyperosmolarity in patients with dry eye, and postulated the measuring of the film's osmolarity as one of the diagnostic milestones of the dry eye. Likewise, osmolarity is one of the diagnostic tests recommended by the committee of the National Eye Institute of the United States of America [15].

Laboratory tests prove that even an increase of 1% in the film's osmolarity is capable of inducing epithelial lesions and alter the normal flow of fluids towards the stroma.

Labbé et al. [16] established that dry eye is a clinical-pathological entity that involves the tear film, the lacrimal glands, and the eyelids, and it produces a large range of physiopathologic alterations where hyperosmolarity is one of the principal factors, assigning it a major diagnostic role. Several authors [17, 18] confirm these reports.

Even though the examining film's osmolarity requires sophisticated equipment and a high-grade qualification to carry it out, we may assess its value by indirectly measuring the concentration of sodium of the film, employing Schirmer's paper strips. Following the method of the sweat test, which consists in measuring the concentration of sodium employing filter paper on the epidermis of children with fibrocystic disease of the pancreas, we evaluate the concentration of sodium which we obtain from tears by humidifying a strip of Whatman 41 paper in the habitual way for Schirmer's test.

Subsequently by using colorimetry we measure sodium concentration in same.

Normally the mean concentration of sodium in the tear film is in the range of 134–170 meq/L; in patients with dry eye concentration, it increases to extreme values (500 meq/L). Later, and employing van't Hoff's formula, we may assess the osmotic pressure of the ion sodium and the indirect index of the film's osmolarity.

$$\text{van't Hoff formula:osmotic pressure} = C \times R \times T \qquad (1)$$

where C is the concentration of the solution, R the universal constant of gases, and T the absolute temperature.

3. Other investigations

In the last decade, numerous authors have highlighted the importance of hyperosmolarity of the tear film in the pathophysiology of dry eye. Lemp et al. [19] and collaborators also grant a significant diagnostic role. Liv et al. [20] relate the instability of the tear film with the increase in osmolarity and give it a fundamental role in the cascade of pathological events that on the ocular surface is capable of generating.

The importance of hyperosmolarity is such that authors such as Hirata et al. [21] suggest that the increased osmolarity of the tear film induces functional and structural lesions of the corneal nerves and neurotoxicity.

In 2010, Mesmer et al. [22] determined that hyperosmolarity is an important factor in the pathophysiology of dry eye.

More recently, the final report of the pathophysiology subcommittee of the TFOS DEWS II [23] concluded that the core mechanism of dry eye is evaporation-induced tear hyperosmolarity that produces a vicious circle (**Figure 1**). When osmolarity rises it causes damage on the ocular surface both directly and by initiating inflammation.

This subcommittee concluded: "tear hyperosmolarity is considered to be the trigger for a cascade of signaling events within surface epithelial cells, which leads to the release of inflammatory mediators and proteases. Such mediators, together with the tear hyperosmolarity itself, are understood to cause goblet cell and epithelial cell loss and damage to the epithelial glycocalyx. Inflammatory mediators from activated Tcells, recruited to the ocular surface, reinforce damage. The net result is the characteristic punctate epitheliopathy of DED and a tear film instability which leads at some point to early tear film breakup. This breakup exacerbates and amplifies tear hyperosmolarity and completes the vicious circle events that lead to ocular surface damage."

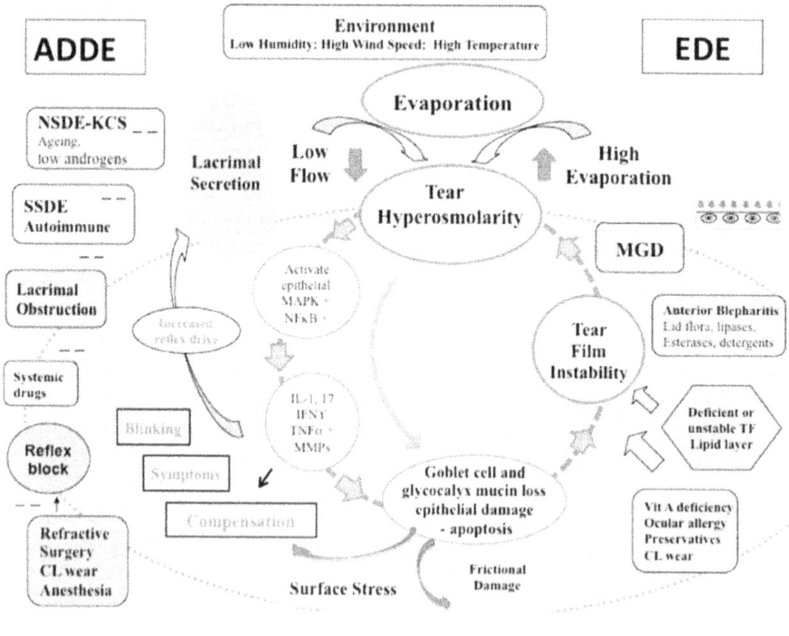

Figure 1.
The vicious circle of dry eye disease. Image obtained from TFOS DEWS II 2017 pathophysiology subcommittee.

4. Conclusions

Undoubtedly, dry eye is nowadays one of the problems most commonly diagnosed by ophthalmologists. The dry eye is a complex multifactor illness of the tear film and of the ocular surface (cornea, conjunctiva, palpebral anexus, glands and nerves) characterized by symptoms of discomfort, vision alterations, and instability of the pre-corneal tear film that may bring about potential damage on the ocular surface. Instability of the film will produce increasing of osmolarity of the tear film, which will trigger epithelium osmotic lesions and inflammation. As these changes take place on the ocular surface, neurophysiologic mechanisms of homeostasis will be altered, which will complicate the process even further, with the cropping up of vicious physiopathologic circuits.

The knowledge of its physiopathologic triggering and its early diagnosis will allow a better management of this pathology. In this sense, evaluation of osmolarity of the tear film in these patients, even if it does not give us an etiologic diagnosis of the disease, does give us an efficient tool to diagnose and evaluate the disease, as its values are directly proportional to the severity of the clinical picture of the dry eye, and is always present in these patients.

Author details

Alejandro Aguilar[1,2*] and Alejandro Berra[3]

1 Ocular Surface Department, Grupo Médico Las Lomas, San Isidro, Buenos Aires, Argentina

2 Ophthalmology Department, Universidad del Salvador, Buenos Aires, Argentina

3 Research Ocular Department, Universidad de Buenos Aires, Buenos Aires, Argentina

*Address all correspondence to: aguilar.alejandrojavier@usal.eduar

IntechOpen

References

[1] Aguilar AJ. Ojo seco, manual sobre fisiopatogenia, diagnóstico y tratamiento. Buenos Aires: Ediciones Científicas Argentinas; 1999. 196 p

[2] Aguilar AJ, Fonseca L, Croxatto OJ. Sjögren syndrome: A comparative study of impression cytology of the conjunctiva and the bucal mucosa, and salivary gland biopsy. Cornea. 1991;**10**:203-206

[3] Gilbard JP, Farris RL. Tear osmolarity and ocular surface disease in keratoconjunctivitis sicca. Archives of Ophthalmology. 1979;**97**:1642-1646

[4] Holly FJ, Patten JT, Dohlman CH. Surface activity determination of aqueous tear components in dry eye patients and normals. Experimental Eye Research. 1977;**24**:479-491

[5] Gilbard JP, Farris RL, Santamaria J. Osmolarity of tear microvolumes in keratoconjunctivitis sicca. Archives of Ophthalmology. 1978;**96**:677-681

[6] Holly FJ, Lamberts DW. Effect of nonisotonic solutions on tear film osmolarity. Investigative Ophthalmology & Visual Science. 1981;**20**:2336-2345

[7] Aguilar AJ, Rodriguez M, Fonseca L, Marré D. El test de Schirmer como método de medida de la concentración de Sodio del film lagrimal y de su osmolaridad en pacientes portadores de ojo seco: Claves de la fisiopatología de la lesión sicca. Archivos de Oftalmología de Buenos Aires. 1993;**68**:189-193

[8] Glasstone D. Elementos de fisicoquímica. Editorial Médico Quirúrgica: Buenos Aires; 1952. 847 p

[9] Fujikawa LS, Foster CS, Gipson IK, Colvin RB. Basement membrane components in healing rabbit corneal epithelial rounds: Immunofluorescence and ultrastructural studies. Journal of Cell Biology. 1984;**98**:128-138

[10] Funderburgh JL, Cintron C, Covington HI, Conrad GW. Immunoanalysis of keratan sulfate proteoglycan from corneal scars. Investigative Ophthalmology & Visual Science. 1988;**29**:116-124

[11] Tseng SCG, Hirst LW, Maumenee AE, Kenyon KR, Sun TT, Green WR. Possible mechanisms for the loss of goblet cells in mucin-deficient disorders. Ophthalmology. 1984;**91**:545-552

[12] Berra A, Berra M. Hyperosmolarity induce nuclear translocation of NF-KB in human conjunctiva epithelial cells. Investigative Ophthalmology & Visual Science. 2005;**46**:4402

[13] Nelson JD. Impression cytology. Cornea. 1988;7(1):71-81

[14] Khanal S, Tomlinson A, McFadyen A, Diaper C, Ramaesh K. Dry eye diagnosis. Investigative Ophthalmology & Visual Science. 2008;**49**(4):1407-1414

[15] Lemp MA. Report of the National Eye Institute/Industry workshop on clinical trials for dry eye. The CLAO Journal. 1995;**21**:221-232

[16] Labbé A, Brignole-Baudouin F, Baudouin C. Ocular surface investigations in dry eye. Journal Français d'Ophtalmologie. 2007;**30**:76-97

[17] Tomlinson A, Khanal s, Ramaesh K, Diaper C, McFadyen A. Tear film osmolarity: Determination of a referent for dry eye diagnosis. Investigative Ophthalmology & Visual Science. 2006;**47**:4309-4315

[18] Berra I, Aguilar AJ, Berra A. Clinical and laboratory tests in patients with dry

eye, allergic conjunctivitis and dry eye plus allergic conjunctivitis. In: ARVO Meeting 1999 May 14

[19] Lemp MA, Bron AJ, Somez B, et al. Clinical utility of objective tests for dry eye disease. American Journal of Ophthalmology. 2011;**151**:792-798

[20] Liv H, Begley C, Chen M. A link between tear instability and hyperosmolarity in dry eye. Investigative Ophthalmology & Visual Science. 2009;**50**:3671-3679

[21] Hirata H, Miserska K, Mafurt C, Rosenblatt M. Hyperosmolar tears induce functional and structural alterations of corneal nerves: Electrophysiological and anatomical evidence toward neurotoxicity. Investigative Ophthalmology & Visual Science. 2015;**56**(13):8125-8140

[22] Mesmer EM, Bulgen M, Kampik A. Hyperosmolarity of the tear film in dry eye syndrome. Developments in Ophthalmology. 2010;**45**:129-138

[23] Bron A et al. TFOS DEWS II pathophysiology report. The Ocular Surface. 2017;**15**:438-510

Recent Advances in the Effects of Various Surgical Methods on Tear Film after Pterygium Surgery

Juan Wang

Abstract

Pterygium is a common ocular disorder with a high prevalence. Surgical resection is the main method of treating pterygium. Recurrence rate of traditional surgical methods such as simple excision of pterygium is high. In recent years, amniotic membrane transplantation, autologous limbal stem cell transplantation, application of mitomycin (MMC) and some other methods become commonly used. Autologous limbal stem cell transplantation is being most widely used. Pterygium has a close relationship with dry eye, and dry eye is one of the important reasons for its recurrence. Different surgical methods have different effects on postoperative tear film. This review will summarize the recent points.

Keywords: pterygium, surgical methods, tear film, dry eye

1. Introduction

Dry eye is a type of disease caused by tear film instability and/or ocular surface damage, which results in eye discomfort and visual dysfunction [1]. The etiology and pathogenesis of dry eye are complicated. Epidemiological studies have shown that there is a positive correlation between pterygium and dry eye [2], and usually accompanied with tear film dysfunction, which is associated with pterygium hyperplasia, irregular, and non-smooth ocular surface. Surgical resection is the main treatment for pterygium which can repair the ocular surface and improve tear film function and reduce dry eye symptoms [3]. It found that different surgical methods of pterygium have different recurrence rates and different tear film function changes [4]. Now, we will summarize the changes of tear film function after different surgical methods of pterygium.

2. Simple excision of pterygium

It reported that the stability of the tear film after pterygium resection is reduced, and dry eye syndrome occurs in severe cases [5]. Compared with preoperative, the tear break-up time (BUT) was significantly prolonged for 1 month after scleral exposure with simple pterygium excision. Tear-ferning test showed a significant increase in normal crystallization ratio, and conjunctival imprint cytology showed a significant increase in goblet cell density. Therefore, they thought that tear function in patients with primary pterygium improves after pterygium excision, which indicates that pterygium has a close relationship with dry eye [6]. However, there was other studies concluded that pterygium removal may not have any effect on Schirmer's test results and tear BUT 1-month post- surgery [7]. Paton observed that a pterygium is further exacerbated by elevation of the pterygium head, dryness, and delle formation [8]. Pterygium excision can partly restore the tear functions into normal state in patients with pterygium which may be due to the increasing density of the conjunctival goblet cell and the recovery of mucus secretion [9]. Simple excision of pterygium is a traditional surgical method, but the recurrence rate is as high as 24–89% [10], and it is currently less applied.

3. Pterygium excision combined with autologous conjunctival transplantation

Kilic et al. [11] investigated the effects of pterygium excision using the limbal conjunctival autografting technique on the tear function tests in 14 eyes of 13 patients. Since no difference was found in the Schirmer and tear BUT tests at 1 and 6 months postoperative versus preoperative. Shortened BUT and the reduced length of Schirmer test after the removal of pterygium combined with autologous conjunctival transplantation are related to the number of operations, the size of the scleral exposed surface, the thickness of the graft, and the location of the graft. Large removal of the nasal conjunctiva intraoperatively, too large conjunctival graft, and the location too close to the dome or too deep can all lead to shortened BUT, reduced tear secretion test length, and prone to dry eye syndrome [12]. Some authors [13] have found that compared with the opposite healthy eyes, the BUT and mucus fern test (MFT) in the eyes with pterygium were significantly different before the operation ($p < 0.05$). The results of the BUT and MFT in the eyes with pterygium were significantly different before and 4 weeks after the operation ($p < 0.05$). The BUT was prolonged and the ratio of normal crystallization in the MFT increased. Tear functions were abnormal in the eyes with pterygium. Pterygium excision combined with conjunctival autograft transplantation can partially restore the tear film function into normal state, and the tear film function was stable 4 weeks after surgery. Zeng et al. [14] compared the recurrence rates after pterygium excision combined with autologous conjunctiva and amniotic membrane transplantation. After 1 year follow-up, the results showed that the combined autologous conjunctival transplantation group was lower than the amniotic membrane transplantation group, and the difference was statistically significant ($p < 0.05$). No statistically significant difference was observed between the two groups in postoperative tear film BUT ($p > 0.05$).

4. Pterygium excision combined with autologous limbal stem cell transplantation

The lack of stem cells at the neck of pterygium [15] provides a theoretical basis for the treatment of pterygium excision combined with limbal stem cell transplantation. Because of the low recurrence rate after excision of pterygium combined with autologous limbal stem cell transplantation [16], it is widely used. Zhang et al. [17] compared the therapeutic effects of recurrent pterygium treated by limbal stem cell autograft transplantation and amniotic membrane transplantation. After the follow-up of 6–24 months, the recurrence rate was 3.03% in limbal stem cell autograft transplantation group, and 22.86% in amniotic membrane transplantation group. There was statistical significant difference between two groups ($p < 0.05$). The average epithelial recovering time of corneal wound was 4.73 and 6.38 days in two groups, the difference was significant (p < 0.05). Limbal stem cells autograft transplantation can decrease the recurrent rate and improve epithelial recovering time of corneal wound. It is an ideal method of recurrent pterygium surgery. It was shown that pterygium excision combined with limbal stem cell transplantation has less effect on tear film function than traditional pterygium excision, and the incidence of dry eye is lower [18]. Other authors [19] compared the incidence of dry eye after the operation of pterygium excision combined with autologous limbal stem cell transplantation and amniotic membrane transplantation. They showed that patients with primary pterygium treated with autologous limbal stem cell transplantation can improve the tear film stability in the early postoperative period and reduce the incidence of dry eye. However, the long-term effects of the two surgical methods and the dry eye are not obvious. Clinically, the surgical method should be reasonably selected according to the actual situation of the patient. Tear film stability of pterygium excision combined with limbal stem cell transplantation is better compared with pterygium excision combined with amniotic membrane transplantation at early postoperative. Patients bear mild symptoms of dry eye [20]. Deng et al. [21] observed the situations of different surgical methods on dry eyes in patients with pterygium excision combined transplantation. Group A underwent pterygium excision combined large autologous conjunctival flap transplantation; group B underwent pterygium excision combined with small conjunctival flap; and group C underwent pterygium excision combined with small conjunctival flap with autologous limbal stem cell. Repair of postoperative corneal epithelium, tear film BUT, and questionnaire of ocular surface disease index (OSDl) preoperation and 1, 3 months postoperation were observed among three groups, which caused the situation of dry eyes by pterygium and pterygium excision were evaluated. They concluded that pterygium excision combined with small conjunctival flap and autologous limbal stem cell shows quickly corneal epithelium recover and low dry eye ratio. Jin et al. [22] investigated the effect of pterygium excision combined with autologous corneal limbus stem cells transplantation on lacrimal film recovery between primary and recurrent pterygium. About 1 week after operation, both groups appeared dryness and shortened BUT, which was more serious in recurrent pterygium group (p < 0.05); there was no significant difference in Schirmer I test between two groups. One month after operation only recurrent pterygium group appeared dryness and shortened BUT compared with primary pterygium group, which was nearly recovered (p < 0.05). Results showed that the recovery of tear stability and lacrimal secretion was poorer in recurrent pterygium than in primary pterygium, which partly explains high recurrence rate of recurrent pterygium. A study [23] suggested that pterygium excision combined with limbal stem cell transplantation can provide a healthy source of epithelial cells. The damaged corneal epithelial surface is repaired, and the limbal anatomy and physiological reconstruction are obtained by the proliferation and differentiation of stem cells and the centripetal repair of cells. Flatter graft makes smoother surface, and the tear film stability is better. In contrast, other authors [24] suggest corneal limbal conjunctival autograft combined with pterygium excision yields sound long-term efficacy and a low recurrence rate than pterygium excision with exposed sclera, and induces only mild damage on the ocular surface. No statistically significant differences are observed between the two groups regarding postoperative tear film BUT.

5. Pterygium excision combined with amniotic membrane transplantation

Amniotic membrane is a thin and transparent membrane in the placenta. It has no blood vessels and lymphatic vessels. It contains a variety of cytokines, which can effectively reduce inflammation, promote wound healing, and anti-fibrosis [25]. The recurrence rate of pterygium excision combined with amniotic membrane transplantation was significantly lower than that of single pterygium excision group [26]. Pterygium excision combined with amniotic membrane transplantation mainly inhibits fibroplasia in the operation area, inhibits leukocyte activation, reduces inflammatory reaction, reduces scar formation, inhibits vascularization, and prevents recurrence of pterygium [27]. Yao [28] compared tear BUT and Schirmer I test at preoperatively, 1, 3 months postoperatively between simple pterygium excision group and pterygium excision combined with amniotic membrane transplantation group, and ocular surface temperature and dry eye symptom score were taken at 2 months after operation. Pterygium excision combined with amniotic membrane transplantation can effectively improve the dry eye, which is conducive to the stability of tear film function. Some authors [29] compared two surgical methods (pterygium excision combined with conjunctival flap transplantation and pterygium excision combined with amniotic membrane transplantation) on tear function. BUT and Schirmer I were shortened on both groups at 1 and 3 months postoperation, and the differences were significant ($p < 0.05$). Pterygium excision affects tear film function at the early postoperative stage. Tear film function returns to preoperative levels 3 months after surgery. Influence of pterygium excision combined with amniotic membrane transplantation on function of the tear film is less than that of pterygium excision combined with conjunctival flap transplantation at early postoperative stage. Amniotic membrane transplantation can limit fibrosis of the sub-conjunctival tissue, improve the success rate of surgery, and reduce the incidence of postoperative dry eye. The reason is the basement membrane surface of the amniotic membrane and the fibroblasts of the conjunctiva stimulate the differentiation of conjunctival goblet cells, keeping the conjunctiva and cornea of the postoperative patients moist, reducing the incidence of dry eye [30].

6. Application of MMC in the treatment of pterygium excision

MMC is an anti-tumor antibiotic isolated from the filtrate of Streptomyces cephalosporin. It inhibits the synthesis of DNA, RNA, and protein and is radiomimetic in many of its actions [31]. It could reduce tissue adhesions and scar formation that has been widely adopted in pterygium surgery to lower the recurrence rate [32]. The purpose of the use of MMC as an adjunctive treatment is to prevent the recurrence of pterygium after the surgery [33]. It has been reported that the wound tissue has not been completely repaired within 2 weeks after pterygium resection. Local use of MMC is prone to lead to ischemic necrosis of wound tissue, especially for patients with bulbar conjunctival flap transplantation [34]. Research [35] has shown that pterygium excision with a free conjunctival autograft combined with intraoperative low-dose MMC is a safe and effective technique in pterygium surgery. MMC can prevent vascular regeneration in the surgical field, prevent fibroblast proliferation and scar formation, and reduce the recurrence rate after pterygium surgery. Intraoperative administration of mitomycin C at 0.05% is safe and effective in preventing pterygium recurrences [36]. Gao et al. [37] compared the clinical efficacy of treatment on recurrent pterygium using different concentration MMC in the pterygium excision operation combined with the corneal limbal stem cell autografting. In their study, complications are corneal edema, corneal ulcer, and conjunctival flap infection. Scleral necrosis occurs in 0.2–4.5% of patients, and higher risk is linked to adjunctive use of MMC, especially more concentrated or repeated doses [38]. It was reported that a case of corneoscleral melt that occurred 50 years after resection of pterygium with postoperative administration of MMC [39]. The application of 0.2 mg/ml MMC during operation for 3 minutes could effectively control fiber hyperplasia of conjunctivas and there are no complications on cornea and sclera [40]. Study [41] shows that the dry eye symptoms, basic tear secretion and BUT values of the MMC group are significantly better than the simple pterygium excision group. The difference between the two groups is statistically significant ($p < 0.05$). Therefore, it is believed that the treatment of pterygium excision combined with MMC has little effect on the stability of tear film and the secretion of basic tears, and the cure rate is high, which is an effective method for treating pterygium [42]. There is no significant difference in the cure rate and recurrence rate between pterygium excision combined with MMC and pterygium excision combined with autologous limbal stem cell transplantation ($p > 0.05$), both of which can effectively treat primary pterygium, but pterygium excision combined with MMC treatment will not destroy the ocular surface microenvironment, and the operation is easy to master, which is worthy of clinical promotion [43]. However, some studies have shown that the use of 0.2 g/L MMC in the treatment of simple pterygium excision showed signs of significant improvement in ocular surface environment early after surgery, and patients who use 0.29/L MMC are observed obvious ocular surface damage, keratinization of epithelial cells, loss of normal cuboid morphology, loose connection between cells, increased cell gap, increased nuclear-to-plasma ratio, and marked decrease in goblet cell density in analyzed area 3 months after surgery [44].

7. Other surgical methods

By combining autologous corneal limbal stem cell transplantation with conjunctival flap and amnion transplantation, the barrier between corneal epithelium and conjunctival epithelium is maintained and the invasion of foreign conjunctival tissue is prevented, so that the recurrence of pterygium and relevant complications are reduced [45]. The operation of transplantation of amniotic membrane and limbal stem cells can further reduce the postoperative recurrence rate [46]. Tear function is abnormal in patients with recurrent pterygium. The tear functions in patients with recurrent pterygium can improve significantly after combined surgery, restore the cornea stem cells and cohesion margin health conjunctival, and promote the ocular surface reconstruction perfect [47]. Tear film stability of pterygium excision combined with limbal stem cell and amniotic membrane transplantation is better than that of pterygium excision combined with limbal stem cell transplantation or amniotic membrane transplantation in early postoperative stage, but the forward performance and severity of xerophthalmia after surgical treatment of pterygium are about the same. Operation method should be chosen according to the patient's condition [48].

8. Summary

Pterygium is a common ocular surface disease, and the prevalence rate is high. The main treatment method is surgical resection. The recurrence rate and incidence of postoperative dry eye after traditional simple pterygium resection is high. The recurrence rate and the incidence of dry eye of pterygium excision combined with autologous limbal stem cell transplantation is low, so it is most widely used currently. The healthy conjunctival tissue will not be damaged in combined amniotic membrane transplantation which provides conditions for glaucoma filtration surgery. Combined use of low concentration of MMC can effectively reduce the recurrence rate of pterygium, easy to operate, but there are risks of long-term complications such as scleral lysis. Amniotic membrane transplantation combined with autologous limbal stem cell transplantation can reduce the recurrence rate of pterygium and recurrent pterygium, and has little effect on the tear film. The surgical method can be selected according to the actual situation of pterygium patients.

Author details

Juan Wang
Department of Ophthalmology, Tianjin Jinghai Hospital, Tianjin, China

*Address all correspondence to: wangjuan1982122@sina.com

IntechOpen

References

[1] Chinese Medical Association Ophthalmology Branch Corneal Disease Group. Dry eye clinical diagnosis and treatment expert consensus (2013). Chinese Journal of Ophthalmology. 2013;**49**(1):73-75

[2] Lee AJ, Lee J, Saw SM, et al. Prevalence and risk factors associated with dry eye symptoms: A population based study in Indonesia. The British Journal of Ophthalmology. 2002;**86**(12):1347-1351

[3] Wen XF, Ke M. Comparison among different surgical treatments for recurrent pterygium: A systematic review. Chinese Journal of Evidence-Based Medicine. 2012;**12**(11):1379-1384

[4] Türkyilmaz K, Öner V, Sivem MS, et al. Effect of pterygium surgery on tear osmolarity. Journal of Ophthalmology. 2013;**2013**:863498

[5] Esquenazi S. Autogenous lamellar scleral graft in the treatment of scleral melt after pterygium surgery. Graefe's Archive for Clinical and Experimental Ophthalmology. 2007;**245**(12):1869-1871

[6] Li M, Zhang M, Lin Y, et al. Tear function and goblet cell density after pterygium excision. Eye (London). 2007;**21**(2):224-228

[7] Kampitak K, Tansiricharemkul W, Leelawongtawun W. A comparison of precorneal tear film pre and post pterygium surgery. Journal of the Medical Association of Thailand. 2015;**98**(Suppl):S53-S55

[8] Paton D. Pterygium management based upon a theory of pathogenesis. Transactions –American Academy of Ophthalmology and Otolaryngology. 1975;**79**:603-612

[9] Li M, Lin YS, Zhang M, et al. Tear functions in patients with pterygium before and after pterygial excision. Chinese Journal of Practical Ophthalmology. 2004;**22**(9):701-705

[10] Kaufman SC, Jacobs DS, Lee WB, et al. Options and adjuvants in surgery for pterygium: A report by the American Academy of ophthalmology. Ophthalmology. 2013;**120**(1):201-208

[11] Kilic A, Gorier B. Effect of pterygium excision by limbal conjunctival auotografting on tear function tests. Annals of Ophthalmology. 2006;**38**(3):235-238

[12] Wei Y, Chen LP, Zhang GF, et al. Causes of dry eye after pterygium excision combined with autologous conjunctival transplantation. Chinese Journal of Practical Ophthalmology. 2002;**20**(6):456-457

[13] Wang S, Jiang B, Gu Y. Changes of tear film function after pterygium operation. Ophthalmic Research. 2011;**45**(4):210-215

[14] Zeng RP, Liang XQ, Wang GP. The comparison of the recurrence rates after pterygium excision combined with conjunctiva and with amnion transplantation. Chinese Journal of Ocular Trauma and Occupational Eye. 2016;**38**(1):39-41

[15] Liu X, Xiao Y, Sheng CJ, et al. A pathological studies on the limbal stem cells in the cervical pterygium. Chinese Journal of Practical Ophthalmology. 2003;**21**(7):499-501

[16] Zhang XF, Fu XY, Yin YC. Long-term follow-up on the recurrence rate of three surgical techniques for pterygium. Chinese Journal of Ocular Trauma and Occupational Eye Disease. 2016;**38**(2):96-99

[17] Zhang Q, Xiang ZY. Compare the effects of recurrent pterygium treated

by limbal stem cell transplantation and amniotic membrane transplantation. Chinese Journal of Practical Ophthalmology. 2006;**24**(5):505-507

[18] Lin JN, Yu L. Clinical comparative analysis of dry eye caused by two kinds of primary pterygium surgery. Yi Yao Qian Yan. 2014;(10):218-219

[19] Fan WJ, Zhao F, Zhao GY, et al. Clinical analysis of dry eye caused by two surgical procedures in primary pterygium surgery. Zhong Wai Yi Xue Yan Jiu. 2016;**14**(36):35-36

[20] Yue H, Ren QJ, Gu SY, et al. Clinical observation of tear film stability on two types of surgical methods for treamlent of pterygiilm. Chinese Journal of Practical Ophthalmology. 2012;**30**(7):823-825

[21] Deng FZ, Kuang GP. Clinical observation of different surgical methods on dry eyes in patients with pterygium excision combined transplantation. International Eye Science. 2015;**15**(5):914-916

[22] Jin J, Xu GX, Zhang J, et al. Lacrimal film recovery following autologous corneal limbus stem cells transplantation for treatment of primary and recurrent pterygium. Zhongguo Zuzhi Gongcheng Yanjiu. 2011;**15**(27):5127-5130

[23] Ren XQ. Clinical observation of pterygium excision combined with limbal stem cell transplantation. Journal of Clinical and Experimental Medicine. 2007;**6**(12):109

[24] Yang Y, Pi M, Xu F. Observation of long-term efficacy of corneal limbal conjunctival autografts in microscopy treatments of pterygium. Eye Science. 2013;**28**(2):73-78

[25] Fan WJ, Yang ZM, Deng L, et al. Basic study on the development of amniotic membrane and its application. Chinese Journal of Reparative and Reconstructive Surgery. 2006;**20**(1):65-68

[26] Zhuang SJ, Lei SC, Cai GH. Comparison of three different surgical excision of pterygium. Journal of Clinical Ophthalmology. 2011;**19**(2):168-170

[27] Gao Y, Jiang Y, Jiang L, et al. Clinical observation of amniotic membrane transplantation for treatment of pterygium. Chinese Journal of Ophthalmology and Otorhinolaryngology. 2005;**5**(5):316

[28] Yao JF. Effect of pterygium excision combined with amniotic membrane transplantation for tear film function. International Eye Science. 2017;**17**(5):1002-1004

[29] Dong JY, Zhang HJ, Huo M, et al. Clinical observation of the dry eye after the different surgical methods for pterygium. Chinese Journal of Practical Ophthalmology. 2014;**32**(8):1015-1018

[30] Jain S, Rastogi A. Evaluation of the outcome of anmiotic membrane transplantation for ocular surface reconstruction in symblepharon. Eye. 2004;**18**(12):1251-1257

[31] Frucht-Pery J, Siganos CS, Ilsar M. Intraoperative application of topical mitomycin-C for pterygium surgery. Ophthalmology. 1996;**103**:674-677

[32] Kunitomo N, Mori S. Studies on the pterygium. Part 4: A treatment of the pterygium by mitomycin-C instillation. Survey of Ophthalmology. 1963;**67**:601-607

[33] Kam KW, Belin MW, Young AL. Monitoring corneal densities following primary pterygium excision with adjuvant topical mitomycin-c application—An observational study of corneal scar changes. 2015;**34**(5):530-534

[34] Yao DQ. Two cases of conjunctival and scleral necrosis caused by mitomycin C. Chinese Journal of Ophthalmology. 1999;2:90

[35] Frucht-Pery J, Raiskup F, Ilsar M, et al. Conjunctival autografting combined with low-dose mitomycin C for prevention of primary pterygium recurrence. American Journal of Ophthalmology. 2006;**141**(6):1044-1050

[36] Rodriguez JA, Ferrari C, Hernández GA.Intraoperative application of topical mitomycin C 0.05%for pterygium surgery. Boletín de la Asociación Médica de Puerto Rico. 2004;**96**(2):100-102

[37] Gao L, Ai M. Comparison of different concentration mitomycin C in the treatment of recurrent pterygium. International Eye Science. 2015;**15**(2):359-360

[38] Ti S, Tan D. Tectonic corneal lamellar grafting for severe scleral melting after pterygium surgery. Ophthalmology. 2003;**110**:1126-1136

[39] Kondo A, Mimura T, Goto M, et al. Letter to the editor: Corneoscleral melt 50 years after excision of pterygium. Open Ophthalmology Journal. 2017;**11**:47-50

[40] Ren HY, Xu YQ, Wu BY, et al. An experimental and clinical research of mitomycin during operation to treat pterygium. Chinese Ophthalmic Research. 2001;**19**(3):273-275

[41] Chen YL, Lu YM, Zhou YQ, et al. Clinical observation and comparative analysis of different treatment methods for the treatment of pterygium. World Health Digest Medical Periodieal. 2013;**10**(16):210-211

[42] Ye WM. Clinical exploration of ocular surface changes after treatment of pterygium excision combined with mitomycin for pterygium. China Medicine and Pharmacy. 2013;**3**(12):199-200

[43] Ji L. Clinical analysis of pterygium excision combined with mitomycin C and combined autologous limbal stem cell transplantation for the treatment of primary pterygium. Acta Academiae Medicinae Xuzhou. 2016;**36**(11):765-766

[44] Liu JR, Li XM, Wang W. Clinical observation of therapeutic efficacy and study of conjunctival impression cytology after pterygium surgery. Chinese Journal of Ophthalmology. 2010;**46**(4):323-327

[45] Zhao X. Autologous corneal limbal stem cell transplantation with conjunctival flap combined with amnion transplantation in treatment of recurrent pterygium. International Eye Science. 2004;**4**(2):354-355

[46] Liu SQ, Zhang JS, Hou ZJ. Curative effect of recurrent pterygium using stem cells of limbus of cornea combined amniotic membrane transplantation. Journal of Practical Preventing Blind. 2006;**11**(4):145-147

[47] Yu M, Xu L. Ocular surface functions reconstruction after joint surgery in patients with recurrent pterygium. Yiyao Qianyan. 2012;**2**(14):44-45

[48] Li L, Yue H, Zhou Q, et al. Xerophthalmia after three surgical methods for treatment of pterygium. China Journal of Modern Medicine. 2016;**26**(15):131-135

Chapter 5

Molecular Genetics of Keratoconus: Clinical Implications

Yu Meng Wang and Calvin C.P. Pang

Abstract

Occurrence of keratoconus is pan-ethnic with reported prevalence ranging widely from 1:400 to about 1:8000, higher in Asian than Western populations. Its genetics is complex with undefined pattern of inheritance. Familial traits are also known. More than 50 gene loci and 200 variants are associated with keratoconus, some through association studies with quantitative traits of cornea features including curvature and central thickness. Environmental, behavioral, and epigenetic factors are also involved in the etiology, likely interactively with genetic susceptibility. Regardless of sex and age of disease onset, clinical courses and responses to treatment vary. Keratoconus is a major cause of cornea transplantation and is potentially blinding. Currently collagen cross-linking provides effective treatment although responses from some patients can be unpredictable with complications. Early diagnosis is vital to obtain good treatment outcome, but in many patients early signs and symptoms are not obvious. While there are potential biomarkers, reliable pre-symptomatic detection and prediction of treatment response may require multitude of gene variants, cornea properties, and external risk factors.

Keywords: keratoconus, genetic markers, clinical implications

1. Introduction

Keratoconus is a progressive corneal disorder involving cone-shaped protrusion and thinning of the central or paracentral cornea, leading to various degrees of visual impairment including astigmatism and even to blindness [1]. Occurrence is usually bilateral but asymmetric between the two eyes, resulting in lopsided visual dysfunction and photophobia with asymmetric progressions and severities of the two eyes in some patients. Many patients started with disease in one eye. Precise age of disease onset is hard to be determined, but it is known to occur mostly in late teenage to early adulthood. Keratoconus is a major cause of visual impairment in young adults in most populations [2]. In one early study, 41% of the keratoconus patients were unilateral at the time of diagnosis [3]. Clinical symptoms and signs range from mild subclinical "forme fruste" or suspect keratoconus to severe and progressive form [4]. In advanced keratoconus, patients may have a v-shaped indentation of the lower eyelid on downgaze caused by a large protuberant cone [5]. Other complications may include apical thinning and irregular astigmatism. Corneal scar and even perforation can happen. Blindness is the eventual consequence to some patients.

The underlying histopathology include reductions in epithelial and stromal keratocytes and collagen contents [6] with degradations of corneal membranes and extracellular matrix. Abnormal mitochondrial functions causing cell death and deranged lipid metabolism are associated with stromal degeneration and disrupted epithelial integrity [7]. The direct causes of pathology are not known. The molecular mechanism of keratoconus has not been identified. Since it is a progressive disease, early detection is important for appropriate treatment in order to avoid serious consequence. A protocol to identify "high-risk" individuals and genetic testing for pre-symptomatic diagnosis would be exceeding helpful.

2. Multi-factorial etiology

The etiology is complex and elusive, affected by interactive environmental and genetic factors [8]. There is association of developmental keratoconus with allergic diseases, eczema, asthma, and hay fever [9, 10]. Contact lens, excessive ultraviolet light, and persistent eye rubbing are risk factors [11, 12] but with no proven and direct cause-and-effect relationships. Links with systemic diseases have been reported [13], including Ehlers-Danlos syndrome and Down syndrome [14]. In an Italian family with osteogenesis imperfecta, which is a connective tissue disorder caused by defects in genes encoding type 1 collagen, ocular features of keratoconus were detected [15]. In Leber congenital amaurosis (LCA), keratoconus has been reported in patients from Pakistan [16, 17], Israel [18], and Australia [19], while LCA itself also features severe retinal dystrophy leading to vision loss. But reported studies are not consistent. In 233 Chinese keratoconus patients in Qingdao located in northern China, 20 (0.86%) of them had had Down syndrome [20]. However, no keratoconus was found in 140 Down syndrome children in Hong Kong in southern China [21] nor in 60 Malaysian [22] or 123 Korean children with Down syndrome [23].

There is currently no causative gene known for keratoconus that causes disease directly [24]. A repertoire of susceptibility genes has been identified with about 200 polymorphisms in more than 50 genes or loci that confer genetic risk to keratoconus [24]. But the available genetic information is insufficient to establish the genetic architecture of keratoconus. No specific pathways have been confirmed. There are, however, clinical implications from studying the keratoconus associated genes. Evidences are in collections for establishment of polygenic risk marker.

3. Timely diagnosis for treatment

Onset of disease is difficult to be determined. Very often patients are not aware of visual symptoms until later stage where ocular discomfort and vision dysfunction becomes obvious. On presentation, slit lamp is capable to detect Fleisher's ring, Vogt's striae, central or paracentral stromal thinning, corneal hydrops and central scarring. But under the slit lamp, early signs are always not obvious [5]. More sophisticated investigative technologies of keratometry, corneal topography and optical coherence tomography provide more sensitive and reliable detection of early keratoconus features on the corneal surface, thickness and curvature. Corneal biomechanical properties can now be evaluated by non-tomographical Scheimpflug imaging and non-tomographical technologies, which are capable to differentiate normal, forme fruste, and keratoconus eyes [25]. In some patients subclinical conditions can be detected [26].

Currently there is no complete cure for keratoconus. At the early stage, vision is usually correctable by spectacles or contact lens. Semi-circular plastic inserts as intrastromal corneal ring segments help reduce astigmatism [27, 28]. However, cornea transplantation is required for severe and progressive keratoconus, which is a major cause for cornea transplantations in many countries [29]. Different types of keratoplasty have been conducted for kerotoconus, penetrating keratoplasty, epikeratoplasty, and deep anterior lamellar keratoplasty (DALK). The latter has the advantage of endothelium preservation [30]. In recent years collagen crosslinking (CXL) has been proved to be safe and effective, in inhibiting, halting, or even reverting to some extent keratoconus progression in a high proportion of patients once correctly diagnosed [31]. There has been decrease in keratoplasty after the advent of collagen crosslinking CXL combines ultraviolet irradiation light and a photosensitizer, such as riboflavin, to strengthen the inter- and intra- crosslinks in the cornea. In 2016 the US Food and Drug Administration (FDA) approved the use of riboflavin and UV for progressive keratoconus by corneal collagen cross-linking [http://avedro.com/press-releases/avedro-receives-fda-approval/]. Over the years, the CXL procedure has been vigorously studied and improved [32, 33]. Meanwhile, for the most effective treatment with best visual outcome, accurate and early detection is mandatory [34]. Younger patients, especially those with a steep maximum keratometry, are at higher risk of disease progression than older patients. The younger the age of the patient, the better is the treatment effect, according to a recent systematic review and meta-analysis involving 11,529 eyes [35]. Early or asymptomatic diagnosis is therefore vital. Recent advances in ophthalmic tomographic imaging and determination of dynamic properties have enabled reliable diagnosis based on early signs [25, 35]. Often, most patients are presented late for ophthalmic consultation and investigations. Prior patients' awareness or notifications of signs and symptoms, genetic testing, if available, would provide diagnosis before symptoms surface [36].

4. Epidemiology and ethnic variations

Occurrence of keratoconus is pan-ethnic and global with a wide range of prevalence traditionally reported from 50 to 230 per 100,000 [1, 3, 37, 38]. A recent meta-analysis of 29 studies up to June 2018 from 15 countries involving over 50 million subjects reported a global prevalence of 138 per 100,000 [39]. There are obvious ethnic variations. For whites the prevalence had been estimated to be 50 in 100,000 [1], whereas blacks and Latinos have approximately 50 percent higher risk of having keratoconus than whites [13]. Asians have higher incidence and prevalence, as well as earlier onset and faster progression than other ethnicities [13, 40].

4.1 Ethnic diversities

In the USA, the overall prevalence was estimated to be 54 per 100,000 according to an early report in 1986 [3]. In a 5-year dataset between 1999 and 2003 for Medicare beneficiaries claiming for keratoconus, the average prevalence was 17.5/100,000 [41]. The records included whites, blacks and Hispanics in ethnicities. There were more whites than other races among the claims. In Denmark, the National Patient Registry recorded 86 keratoconus patients per 100,000 during an 11-year period from 1995 to 2005 [42]. In a study in the United Kingdom, the respective prevalence for Asians (mostly Indians) and Caucasians was 229 and 57 per 100,000, respectively, and corresponding age of diagnosis was 22.3 and 26.5 years [43]. Consistent results were reported in two latter studies comparing Pakistanis and Caucasians in the United Kingdom indicating greater prevalence in Asians by 4.4–7.5 times than Caucasians [44, 45]. In the Middle East in an Iranian population, a prevalence of about 25 per 100,000 and age of diagnosis at 27.1 ± 9.3 years were reported [46]. But in a recent study on a rural population in Iran, a very high prevalence of 4000 per 100,000 was found [47]. In a hospital based study in Saudi Arabia, the incidence was 20 per 100,000 in young patients age ranged from 8 to 24 years, with more than half (54%) of patients classified as advanced keratoconus [48]. In India, onset of disease has been reported to happen at a younger age and progresses more rapidly [49]. In a study totaling 5200 Indian patients, the average age of presentation was 21.5 years with 1970 patients (37.9%) having an onset of disease before 20 years of age. The overall prevalence was very high at 5200/100,000 (5.2%) [50]. In a rural population in central India, a slightly lower prevalence of 2300/100,000 was recorded [51]. In huge contrast, the prevalence in Japanese was low: 12 in 100,000 males and 5.6 in 100,000 females [52]. In Chinese, a population based study in Beijing for an elder population of 3468 individuals aged 50–93 years, steep cornea/keratoconus occurred in 33 persons, giving a prevalence of 950 in 100,000 [53]. In this study steep cornea/keratoconus was defined as corneal refractive power equal to or greater than 48 diopters according to optical low-coherence reflectometry. In a study 2 years later in Singapore in people older than 40 years, the prevalence of steep cornea was comparable in Malays (606 in 100,000), Indians (1000 in 100,000), and Chinese (500 in 100,000) (0.5%) (95% CI 0.3–0.8%) [54].

4.2 Basis for ethnic diversities

A summary of reported studies (**Table 1**) shows in general higher prevalence in Asians than Caucasians, with disease started earlier and severe. But occurrence at Japanese is low. There are also vast differences in the same ethnic group. Environmental factors and investigative criteria other than genetics would affect the reported occurrence of keratoconus. The very wide range of keratoconus prevalence and incidence may be a result of non-uniform diagnostic criteria applied in different studies. Another cause may be genetic variations among different ethnic populations. There is a significant role of ethnicity. Hence rigorous, multiethnic, well-organized, and population-based epidemiological studies with large sample sizes for keratoconus are needed. Nevertheless, in addition to ethnicity, currently reported epidemiologic studies indicate that potential causes underlying higher prevalence of keratoconus could be due to a host of factors including geographic locations, ultraviolet irradiation exposure, consanguinity, persistent eye rubbing and atopy. The etiology of keratoconus is complex, involving multi-factorial interactions of genetic, personal, and environmental factors.

Study	Ethnicity	Prevalence	Age at diagnosis	Year of report	Reference
Japan	Japanese	7.6 in 100,000 12 in 100,000 males 5.6 in 100,000 females		2002	[52]
Singapore	Malay Indian Chinese	Steep cornea/keratonconus 606 in 100,000 1,000 in 100,000 500 in 100,000		2014	[54]
China	Chinese Bejing Eye Study, northern China	Steep cornea/keratonconus 950 in 100,000	aged 50–93 years	2012	[53]
India	Indian	2300 in 100,000 5200 in 100,000	53.2±11.3 years 21.5 years	2015,2009	[50], [51]
Iran		25 per 100,000 4000 in 100,000	27.1±9.3 years	2012,2018	[46], [47]
Saudi Arabia	Saudi Arabian	20 in 100,000	17.7 ± 3.6 years for males (range 8–24 years) 19.0±3.8 years for females (range 12–28 years)	2005	[48]
U.K.	Caucasians Indians	57 in 100,000 229 in 100,000	26.5 years 22.3 years	2000	[43]
U.S.A.	Whites and Blacks Whites, Blacks and Hispanics	54 in 100,000 17.5/100,000		1986 2009	[3], [41]

Table 1.
Geographical and ethnical diversities in reported prevalence of keratoconus.

5. Gender differences

Whether males and females have different prevalence is unclear as inconsistent results have been reported [55]. Disease onset in males tend to be earlier and disease progression faster than female patients in both Asian and Western studies, while gender bias has not been consistent [40, 50, 56, 57]. Male and female sex, did not show difference in prevalence, while gender bias have not been consistent in previous reports. In a Japanese cohort of 90 patients, men were diagnosed younger than women [58]. A questionnaire survey of 670 patients in New Zealand also showed male patients were detected at younger ages than females [59]. In a Turkish cohort of 248 patients, there was no gender difference in cornea properties including central cornea thickness and keratometry parameters [56]. In a study in the USA of 1209 patients from 16 clinics, while there was no difference in disease severity according to keratometry or scarring, less women were had have Vogt striae [57]. Female patients in this study had higher mean age than the males. Overall, there was indication that men developed keratoconus earlier, progressed faster and required more serious treatment.

6. Twins and familial segregation

6.1 Twins with keratoconus

As early as 1954 occurrence of keratoconus in both identical twins had been reported [60]. Following twins reports in different ethnic groups, one twin pair was found to show different contrast sensitivities [61]. However, two pairs of Caucasian identical twins both showed similar features clinically and under videokeratography and radial keratotomy, as one pair were at early and the other as later stage [62]. Two pairs of monozygotic twins were found discordant for keratoconus in the USA, one from a hispanic family of Mexican descent and the other Caucasian from England [63], while dissimilarity in phenotype may suggest the absence of genetic involvement. However, natural monozygotic discordance could occur if there was separation of the zygote into two distinct cell masses after fertilization before the start of tissue differentiation. Post-zygotic events that lead to existence of two different cell clones in the early zygote may precede the twinning process. In the Mexican family, 39 members were examined and 5 were suspected for keratoconus by corneal topography. Also, one distant relative was a confirmed keratoconus patient. Corneal topography also revealed one suspect from 59 family members examined in the English family. There could be a genetic component in the keratoconus phenotype in these two families [63]. Of note, more and more concordant twins with keratoconus have been reported, including reported concordance in all 13 monozygotic and 5 dizygotic twins [64].

6.2 Familial linkage

In the Collaborative Longitudinal Evaluation of Keratoconus (CLEK) study in a cohort of 1209 patients mixed in ethnicity in the USA, 829 (69%) white, 240 (20%) black, and 99 (8%) Hispanic, family history of keratoconus was reported in 13.5% of the cases [65]. After follow-up for 8 years, the inheritance patterns were not established [66]. In another study from the USA, more females reported family history than males. But it was unclear whether it was a difference in attitude on reporting or a genuine gender difference in familial link [57]. In the New Zealand study, familial aggregation analysis showed keratoconus familial rate of 23.5% [59]. In Scotland, family history occurred in 5% of 186 white patients [67]. In a report from North India among 120 patients, 6 (5%) had family history [68]. In a review of keratoconus in Asians, family history ranged from 4.4 to 23.5% [40]. Overall, reported family history of keratoconus has widely ranged from 6% up to about 25% [37, 65].

A recent systemic review and meta-analysis on 29 eligible reports from different parts of the world selected from 3996 articles revealed family history as the strongest risk factor (odds ratio 6.42; 95% CI:2.59–10.24) among other established risk factors: eye rubbing (odds ratio 3.09; 95% CI:2.17–4.00), eczema (odds ratio 2.95; 95% CI:1.30–4.59), asthma (odds ratio 1.94; 95% CI:1.30–2.58), and allergy (odds ratio 1.42; 95% CI:1.06–1.79) [69]. Overall, no obvious differences exist in clinical or ophthalmic presentations between familial and sporadic keratoconus. As a genetic disease, keratoconus has shown weak penetrance with variable expressions. While family aggregation and linkage studies showed familial inheritance, the majority of reported keratoconus patients are sporadic.

7. Mapping the keratoconus genes

Candidate gene analysis, family linkage analysis, and more recently genome-wide association study with support by candidate gene association studies and next generation sequencing, have contributed to identification of genetic loci or gene variants that are in association with keratoconus [70]. All are genetic associations. No direct keratoconus causing mutation has been identified.

7.1 Linkage analysis

Single nucleotide polymorphisms (SNPs) and microsatellite markers covering the whole genome have been attempted to find keratoconus loci or even genes in family pedigrees and sib pairs. But even in families, penetrance of keratoconus is low and clinical presentations are variable. A large number of samples have to be available. Vigorous research among various ethnic groups have identified a number of keratoconus loci which are replicable and of maximum LOD score greater than 3, in a collection of 67 sib pair Hispanic families, two-stage genome-wide analysis of 380 microsatellite markers in totally 351 subjects, among them 110 were affected by keratoconus which has led to identification of a multitude of loci in chromosomes *2q, 3p, 4q, 5q31, 5p, 9p, 9q34, 11p, 12p, 14q,* and *17q* [71]. In a collection of 25 Italian families, genome-wide scan of microsatellite markers in 77 affected and 57 unaffected members have mapped chromosomal regions for keratoconus in *5q32-q33; 5q21.2, 14q11.2,* and *15q2.32* [72]. Some of these loci had been replicated or refined in further investigations: *2p24* [73]; *3p14-q13* [74]; *5q14.3-q21.1* [75]; 5q31.1-q35.3 [72]; *13q32* [76]; *16q22.3-q23.1* [77]; and *20q12* [78]. These studies were mostly on European populations. The large number of associated loci exemplified the genetic heterogeneity of keratoconus. No disease-causing mutation has been identified from these loci.

7.2 Genome-wide association studies (GWAS)

Most GWAS in connection with keratoconus were conducted on the two quantitative traits of central corneal thickness (CCT) and corneal curvature (CC). These two are characteristic, but not exclusive, traits of keratoconus, with the corresponding morphological features of central corneal thinning and corneal steepness.

7.2.1 Central corneal thickness (CCT)

There were nine reported GWAS on central corneal thickness (CCT) up to July 2017. They were summarized in an excellent review [70]. All involved meta-analysis in initial and validation cohorts. More than 40 SNPs in 30 genes were reported. The biggest sample size was with totally 13,057 European and 6963 Asian samples, while the primary cohort was comprised of 874 patients and 6085 controls. A multitude of keratoconus associated SNPs in 26 loci was identified. SNP rs9938149 in the *BANP-ZNF469* gene attained GWAS significance of P-value = 2.4×10^{-49}, which was the highest among all reported SNPs [79].

Some of the gene variants were analyzed in keratoconus and control cohorts. Possibly there was ethnic specificity. Rs96067 in COL8A2 was identified in a Singaporean cohort of 2538 Indians and 2542 Malays [80] but not in a separate GWAS study 0f European study subjects with 3931 German and 1418 Dutch study subjects. However, SNPs in *BANP-ZNF469* and COL5A1 were replicated [81]. In a cohort of Australian white study subjects with 933 keratoconus patients and more than 4000 controls, keratoconus susceptibility was detected at the *HGF* locus [82]. The risk factor allele rs3735520 was associated with keratoconus in a Czech cohort of 165 patients and 193 controls [83] and Australian whites of 157 patients and 673 controls [84]. Another study involved two independent cohorts of keratoconus patients, involving 222 Caucasian patients, 687 African Americans, 3324 Caucasian controls and 307 individuals from 70 keratoconus families reported strong association of *Lysyl Oxidase* gene (*LOX*) polymorphisms with keratoconus, with meta P-values of 2.5×10^{-7} and 4.0×10^{-5} for LOX SNPs rs2956540 and rs10519694 respectively [85]. In a meta-analysis of 14 studies comprising 17,803 individuals of European ancestry 44 loci associated with CCT were found, two of them were LTBP1 and WNT10A 42 European specific while the rest occurred also in Asian ethnicities [86].

7.2.2 Corneal curvature (CC)

Six GWAS on corneal curvature (CC) have been reported in multi-ethnic cohorts that contributed to identification of susceptibility genes. Eight SNPs in MTOR/FRAP1 and 7 SNPs in PDGFRA were found in 10,008 samples from three population groups in Singapore: Malays, Chinese and Indians [87]. Another big cohort of 12,660 Asians included Japanese in addition to Malays, Chinese, and Indians, [88] Associations of CMPK1 rs17103186 and RBP3 rs11204213 with CC, and RBP3 rs11204213 with axial length were discovered. In the Avon Longitudinal Study of Parents and Children (ALSPAC) cohort of 2023 individuals of white European descent, rs6554163 in *PDGFRA* was associated with both CC and axial length [89]. In a cohort of 1013 Australian individuals, 1788 twins and their families, CC was associate with rs2114039 near *PDGFRA* and rs2444240 which is 31 kb upstream to *TRIM29*, but not with any SNP at the FRAP1 locus [90]. In totally 15,168 study samples that included Japanese, Chinese or European ethicity, rs10453441 in WNT7B was strongly associated with both CC and axial length [91]. WNT7B rs10453441 is the only SNP associated with both traits of CCT and CC [92]. While these SNPs have no consistent and strong association with keratoconus, an exome sequencing analysis identified a *WNT10A* variant that was associated with corneal thickness and keratoconus [93]. In contrast, a GWAS on direct association of keratoconus patients and controls involving 222 patients and 3324 controls found no GWAS significance of associated gene variants [94].

7.2.3 Other approaches

Apart from corneal morphologic features, a recent GWAS investigated corneal biomechanical properties in an European cohort of 6645 participants and 2384 participants from the British TwinsUK study [36]. The second stage of the association study involved 752 keratoconus patients as compared with 974 British TwinsUK or 13,828 EPIC-Norfolk. The results showed a likely role in development of keratoconus with 5 associated loci in CH, *ANAPC1, ADAMTS8, ADAMTS17, ABCA6*, and *COL6A1* [36].

It is notable that there are a lot more keratoconus genes that are identified through studies on quantitative traits, especially central cornea thickness and cornea curvature, than on direct association with keratoconus against controls (**Figure 1**).

7.3 Candidate genes

Strategies of genomic search for disease genes are essentially free of a hypothesis to find genes or loci with susceptibility to a disease entity or quantitative trait. For keratoconus, mutation analysis in many candidate genes have also been attempted to find disease causative genes, some followed a biological hypothesis and some based on high GWAS significance. More than 50 SNPs in about 20 genes showing association with keratoconus have been studied in various ethnic populations [70, 95]. They include *FOXO1* [96]; ZNF469 [97]; *COL4A4* [98]; *COL4A3* [99]; *VSX1* [100, 101]; *COL5A1* [102]; *MPDZ-NFIB* [102, 103]; *IL1B* [104, 105]; *HGF* [84]; *LOX* [85, 106]; and *IL1RN* [107]. Some of these genes have been studied in many populations with inconsistent results.

7.3.1 VSX1

The *VSX1* (visual system homeobox 1) gene has been regarded as a candidate keratoconus with about 20 missense variants being putatively disease causative [101, 108]. *VSX1* sequence variants have been extensively screened in different populations including Caucasians, Indians, Chinese, Iranians and Koreans. But segregation of *VSX1* missense variants with keratoconus has been inconsistent and there is no confirmed causative mutation in *VSX1* for keratoncous. p.Leu268His (c.803 T > A)

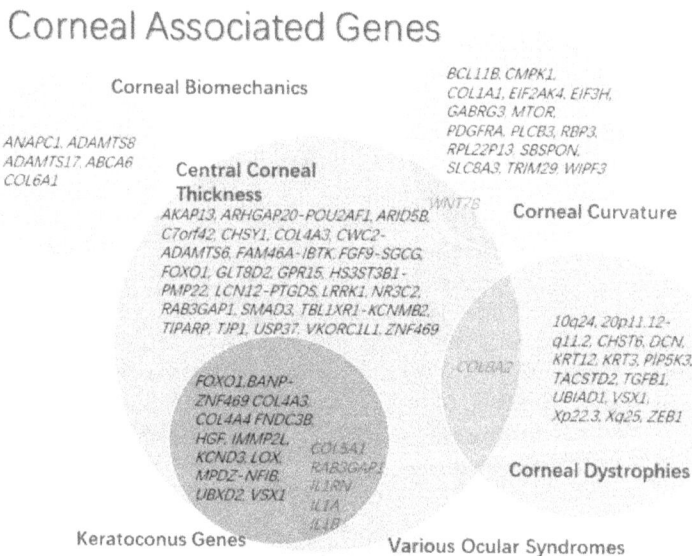

Figure 1.
Cornea associated genes.

was proposed to be foundation mutation as a shared haplotype occurred in 5 Indian keratoconus patients from 2 unrelated families [109]. But it has not been reported in other studies on Indian, Iranian, Korean and other populations.

7.3.2 IL1A and IL1B

The interleukin genes *IL1A* and *IL1B* have been studied in several keratoconus cohorts as they are mediators of keratocyte apoptosis which may occur in corneal injuries that lead to epithelial or endothelial-stromal reorganization as in keratoconus [110, 111]. Screening for *IL1* gene cluster mutations in a Korean cohort of 100 patients and 100 controls identified −31*C (rs1143627) and − 511*T (rs16944) in the *IL1B* promoter posed risk for keratoconus with a combined significance of P = 0.012, OR = 2.38, 95% CI = 1.116-5.05) [104]. Similar association in a Japanese study of 169 patients and 390 controls was reported with a haplotype of −31*C and - 511*T, P = 4.0×10^{-5} and OR = 1.72 [105]. The association was replicated in 115 Han Chinese patients and 101 healthy controls, with significance for −31*C, P > 0.001, OR = 2.86, and P = 0.002, OR = 2.4 for −511*T. SNP IL1A rs2071376 also showed association with P = 0.017, OR = 1.97. The respective ACA haplotype of these 3 promoter SNPs was found to contribute a high risk in this Chinese cohort, P < 0.001, OR = 12.91 [112]. Such statistical significance shows a link of *IL1A* and *IL1B* with keratoconus, and the reported associations are more consistent than other candidate genes. It should be of interest to study the biological effects of these promoter polymorphisms on corneal tissue cells.

7.3.3 MPDZ-NF1B

The *MPDZ* (multiple PDZ domain crumbs cell polarity complex component) and *NFIB* (nuclear factor I B *NF1B*) genes was found to confer risk to keratoconus based on GWAS on central corneal thickness (CCT) of multi-ethnic Asian populations in Singapore. rs1324183 of *MPDZ-NF1B* gave a significance of $P = 8.72 \times 10^{-8}$ [113]. The association was replicated inn Australian Caucasian cohort, P = 0.001, OR = 1 [114]. Further examination of the CCT loci in keratoconus patients from two independent Caucasian cohorts also revealed association rs1324183 for keratoconus, $P = 5.2 \times 10^{-6}$, OR = 1.33 [79]. In a Han Chinese cohort of 210 patients and 191 controls in northern China, the association was p = 0.005, OR = 3.1 [115]. However, no association was found in a Saudi Arabia study of 108 patients and 300 controls [116]. In contrast, very high risk of rs1324183 to keratoconus, $P = 4.30 \times 10^{-4}$ OR = 2.22 was shown after genotyping of 133 patients and 367 controls who are Han Chinese in Hong Kong in southern China [117]. In addition, rs1324183 conferred a higher risk to severe keratoconus (OR = 5.10) than the moderate (OR = 2.05) or mild (OR 2.36) form. There was significant correlation between the risk allele A of rs1324183 with the corneal mechanic parameters of anterior Kf, anterior AvgK, posterior Kf and apex pachymetry, indicating association with corneal thickness and curvature. Therefore rs1324183 has been proposed to be a genetic marker for severity and progression of keratoconus [117]. Taken together, there is no evidence of direct causation to keratoconus by *MPDZ-NF1B*, which, however, does pose susceptibility to development and progression of keratoconus.

7.3.4 COL4A3, COL4A4 and COL5A1

The collagen genes *COL4A3*, *COL4A4* and *COL5A1* are related to corneal collagen structure and development during embryonic development. Its association with keratoconus was first reported in a Slovenia study of white study subjects,

104 patients and 157 controls, with 3 variants, P141L, D326Y, and G895G, in COL4A3 and 5 variants in COL4A4P482S, M1327 V, V1516 V, and F1644F differentiating patients and controls with statistical significance P < 0.005 [118]. Association was replicated in a Greek study [99]. In an Iranian cohort of 112 patients and 150 controls, The COL4A4 RS2229813 (M1327 V) An allele increased keratoconus risk for KC (P = 0.018, OR = 1.5), but COL4A4 RS2228555 (C1516V) showed no association [98].

Another COL4A4 SNP, RS2228557 (F1644F) in 144 patients, 153 controls in Iran, showed a high association (P = 0.0001) [119]. *COL4A4* rs2229813 and RS2228557 are strongly associated with keratonconus in Americans (P = 1.3×10^{-12}, OR = 2.38 and P = 4.5×10^{-7}, OR = 0.54 respectively) [102]. Replication in a Chinese cohort showed weak association [120]. Although *COL4A3* and *COL4A4* plays biological roles in cornea structure and properties, there is no evidence that they directly cause keratoconus.

8. Specific proteins

The pathophysiology of keratoconus is attributed to disruption of the cornea morphology in association with the corneal collagen. A review of published studies on proteins, collagen and risk factors of keratoconus between January 2016 and June 2018 has revealed altered regulations in more than 30 proteins and their genes. They belong to protein families including degradative enzymes, cellular proteases, and collagens [121]. Up- and downregulations of hosts of proteins in corneal epithelium and stroma have been reported in keratoconus, especially different types of collagen and matrix metalloproteinases.

8.1 Collagen

Collagen is the major structural protein in the cornea. Decrease in collagen lamellae and fibers, together with reduced microfibers and fine granules, has been described in keratoconus [122]. Disruption in collagen contents and integrity affect corneal thinning and properties. Reduction of types I, III, and IV, which are major structural proteins in the basement membranes, have been shown in keratoconus [123]. Among the 6 main subtypes of COL4A, which plays important structural and functional roles, COLA4A1 is reportedly downregulated in cornea of keratoconus patients [124]. Expression studies also showed downregulation of many collagen types and subtypes in keratoconus, including COL8A1, COL8A2, COL12A1, COL13A1, COL6A2, COL15A1, and COL18A1 [125–127]. They may be considered for use as biomarkers in keratoconus, [121] but practical protocols and validations are still to be established.

8.2 Matrix metalloproteinases

MMP-1 and MMP-9, are upregulated in corneal tissue and affect collagen properites and dyregulate proteolysis [128]. In a pathways enrichment analysis of 19 keratoconus genes consistently reported as risk genes to keratoconus in 16 studies, interleukin-1 processing and assembly of collagen fibrils are associated with keratoconus pathology [129]. MMPs have been assayed in tears. It is noted that in one study there was no detectable MMP-1 in tears of healthy subjects [130]. Elevations in MMP-1 [131] and MMP-9 levels [132] has been shown in keratoconus tear samples. On study reported correlation between MMP-9 level and disease severity [133]. However, other studies did not find MMP-9 elevation [131, 134].

Inconsistent findings are also reported for MMP-3, MMP-7 and MMP-13 [128]. All in all, there are consistent evidence on elevated MMP-9 levels in keratoconus cornea tissues and tears. Given the important role of MMP-9 in extracellular matrix regulations and corneal inflammation, MMP-9 assay should be useful for monitoring keratoconus treatment. A point-of-care test for MMP-9 in tears has been established for quick and reliable MMP-9 tear essay that facilitates the treatment monitoring [135].

9. Molecular markers

After meta-analysis of 24 eligible studies selected after screening of 668 reports between 1950 and 2016, 16 SNPs in 14 genes/loci were found to be associated with keratoconus out of 53 polymorphisms in 28 genes/loci. Stratification analysis revealed strong association of 8 SNPs in 6 genes/loci with keratoconus in Whites, including *FOXO1* rs2721051, *RXRA-COL5A1* rs1536482, *FNDC3B* rs4894535, *IMMP2L* rs757219 and rs214884, and *BANP-ZNF469* rs9938149, and COL4A4.

rs2229813 and rs2228557 [95]. While they may be potential genetic markers for keratoconus in Whites, there is no further data of validation. Replications in Chinese and Arabic populations [120] revealed weak associations in *COL4A4* rs2229813 and rs2228557, which are strongly associated with keratonconus in Whites with statistical significance of $P = 1.3 \times 10^{-12}$, OR = 2.38 and $P = 4.5 \times 10^{-7}$, OR = 0.54 respectively. In Chinese, another SNP, rs1324183 in *MPDZ-NF1B*, is related to disease severity and corneal biomechanical properties, and may be a potential molecular marker [136].

In a review in 2001 keratoconus was reputed to be an inheritable disease [137]. Since then more evidences of familial links and susceptible genes or loci have been reported as a result of vigorous research in different populations and geographic locations. There are proven genetic and non-genetic risk factors [35]. In a recent

Genes	Variants	Study design	Study population	Keratoconus patients (n)	Controls (n)	P	OR (95%CI)	Reference
HGF and 12 loci	rs3735520 rs17501108 rs3014801	GWAS + Validation	Australia, America	933	4164	0.002 0.0002 0.0004	1.50 (1.15–1.94) 2.33 (1.17–3.69) 2.22 (1.41–3.48)	[82]
3p26-3q21.3.19q13.3 and 12 loci	rs6442095 rs4954018 rs4428642	GWAS + Validation	America	222	3324	6.5×10-8 2.4×10-7 3.4×10-7	1.85 0.5 0.59	[94]
LOX	rs10519694 rs2956540	GWAS + Validation	America	222	3324	2.3×10-5 7×10-5	0.67 0.73	[85]
FOXO1 and FNDC3B	rs2721051 rs4894535	GWAS + Validation	Australia, Northern Ireland and America	874	6085	2.7×10-10 4.9×10-9	1.69 (1.4–1.88) 1.47 (1.29–1.68)	[97]
WNT10A	rs121908120	Exome Sequencing	Australia	621	1580	6.03×10-10		[91]
TFAM ND1 COX1 ND6 POLRMT TFB2M		Mitochondrial genome expression study	Chinese	198	106	3.26×10-3 1.79×10-3 1.54×10-4 4.62×10-3 9.55×10-4 7.88×10-5		[138]
VSX1	c7720c6541 rs8123716	Sanger sequencing	Polish	42	50	0.491 0.278		[139]
TNFα	rs1800629	Case-control Association Study	Pakistan	257	253	<0.001	6.07 (4.08–10.42)	[140]
MPDZ, FOXO1, MAP3K19 RAB3GAP1	rs1324183 rs2721051 rs4954018	Case-control Association Study	Czech	165	193	0.01 0.025 0.047	1.58 (1.10–2.24) 1.72 (1.07–2.77) 1.54 (1.01–2.34)	[141]
VSX1	R13P G160V	Case-control Association Study	Chinese	50	50		R13P in 1 patient G160V in 2 patients none in controls	[142]
	L08H rs6012921 (D105E) rs6050307 (R119I)	Exome Sequencing	Brazilian	73	107	0.121 0.108	L08H in 3 patients 3.86 (0.73–20.5) 2.71 (0.77–9.68)	[144]
TUBA3D	Q11X V68LR*2 c.*2 G>A	Exome Sequencing	Chinese	202	200		Q11X in 1 twins family V68LR*2 in 1 patient c.*2 G>A in 1 patient none in controls	[143]
COL5A3 MPDZ		Exome Sequencing and targeted gene sequencing	Australian	385	396	0.024 0.045	0.54 (0.30–0.96) 0.65 (0.42–0.99)	[145]
CAST	rs4434401	Case-control Association Study	Chinese	120	305	0.037	1.47 (1.02–2.11)	[146]

Table 2.
The keratoconus genes [138–146].

comprehensive review of environmental risk factors and family history, genetic factors are taken to play a role in the etiology of keratoconus [39]. As of today all reported genes for keratoconus, whether mapped by candidate gene strategy or genomic search including GWAS and WES, are susceptibility genes and not causative genes that cause disease directly (**Table 2**). Keratoconus causative genes are still to be identified. As for the reported genes, there is no segregation of gene variants that accounts for higher occurrences of disease. There are also no hotspot variants that are present in a high proportion of patients. Molecular markers for pre- symptomatic detection and risk assessment of keratonocus are still to be established.

10. Genetic implications on treatment

Findings in genetic studies help to delineate the molecular basis of diseases through identification of genes that are causative or susceptible to development of diseases. Investigation of their properties, functions, related pathways and mechanisms throw light on disease pathogenesis. Genetic information also helps to establish genetic markers used for early or even pre-symptomatic diagnosis. Prior to treatment timely detection is extremely important as keratoconus is progressive and the resultant corneal disruptions are hardly curable. With the advent of collagen cross-linking, disease progression can be halted in most patients with some partial recovery of vision. Some patients may respond less favorably and ultimately may require cornea transplantation. Genetic marker, if linked to response to clinical course and treatment, will be exceedingly useful. Over the years in keratoconus vigorous research has been conducted in different ethnic populations in its molecular genetics. However, with the repertoire of associated genes that has been identified at present, no definite genetic marker for diagnosis, risk assessment or prognosis has been established. Further work is warranted.

11. Conclusive remarks and future perspectives

The pathogenesis of keratoconus is heterogeneous and complex. Epidemiological studies showed higher prevalence, earlier onset and greater progression in Asians than Europeans. Both environmental and genetic factors play roles in the etiology and pathogenesis, including age, gender, ocular atopy, eye rubbing, family history, and systemic diseases. While family aggregation and linkage studies indicated genetic abnormality in keratoconus, GWAS and candidate gene studies identified polymorphisms in genes/loci related to the risk of keratoconus. So far there are very few reported big family studies, which should help to identify the keratoconus causative gene. Also, big cohorts are needed to provide sufficient power to differentiate phenotypes and clinical courses of patients for association with genetic factors. Current epidemiological and genetic data are insufficient to provide conclusive evidence to establish the molecular mechanism and genetic markers for keratoconus. Notably, genetic studies on the corneal structure, principally central cornea thickness and cornea curvature have successfully mapped keratoconus genes. Corneal properties, as recently exemplified by a successful GWAS on corneal biomechanical properties [36], should provide a basis for genetic research. Rigorous and large multi-center population-based studies, with age-standardized rates, random sampling, progression follow-ups, and accurate and standardized diagnosis, are warranted for better understanding of pathogenesis of keratoconus and for establishment of genetic markers.

Author details

Yu Meng Wang and Calvin C.P. Pang*
Department of Ophthalmology and Visual Sciences, The Chinese University of
Hong Kong, Hong Kong, China

*Address all correspondence to: cppang@cuhk.edu.hk

IntechOpen

References

[1] Rabinowitz YS. Keratoconus. Survey of Ophthalmology. 1998;**42**(4):297-319

[2] Olivares Jimenez JL et al. Keratoconus: Age of onset and natural history. Optometry and Vision Science. 1997;**74**(3):147-151

[3] Kennedy RH, Bourne WM, Dyer JA. A 48-year clinical and epidemiologic study of keratoconus. American Journal of Ophthalmology. 1986;**101**(3):267-273

[4] Alio JL, Shabayek MH. Corneal higher order aberrations: A method to grade keratoconus. Journal of Refractive Surgery. 2006;**22**(6):539-545

[5] Fan Gaskin JC, Patel DV, McGhee CN. Acute corneal hydrops in keratoconus - new perspectives. American Journal of Ophthalmology. 2014;**157**(5):921-928

[6] Ku JY et al. Laser scanning in vivo confocal analysis of keratocyte density in keratoconus. Ophthalmology. 2008;**115**(5):845-850

[7] Chaerkady R et al. The keratoconus corneal proteome: Loss of epithelial integrity and stromal degeneration. Journal of Proteomics. 2013;**87**:122-131

[8] Sugar J, Macsai MS. What causes keratoconus? Cornea. 2012;**31**(6):716-719

[9] Karseras AG, Ruben M. Aetiology of keratoconus. The British Journal of Ophthalmology. 1976;**60**(7):522-525

[10] Merdler I et al. Keratoconus and allergic diseases among Israeli adolescents between 2005 and 2013. Cornea. 2015;**34**(5):525-529

[11] Hartstein J. Keratoconus that developed in patients wearing corneal contact lenses. Report of four cases. Archives of Ophthalmology. 1968;**80**(3):345-346

[12] Gasset AR, Houde WL, Garcia-Bengochea M. Hard contact lens wear as an environmental risk in keratoconus. American Journal of Ophthalmology. 1978;**85**(3):339-341

[13] Woodward MA, Blachley TS, Stein JD. The association between sociodemographic factors, common systemic diseases, and keratoconus: An analysis of a nationwide heath care claims database. Ophthalmology. 2016;**123**(3):457-465

[14] Robertson I. Keratoconus and the Ehlers-Danlos syndrome: A new aspect of keratoconus. The Medical Journal of Australia. 1975;**1**(18):571-573

[15] Zeri F, Swann PG, Naroo S. Osteogenesis imperfecta and keratoconus in an Italian family. Clinical & Experimental Optometry. 2017;**101**(3):400-403

[16] McKibbin M et al. Genotype-phenotype correlation for leber congenital amaurosis in northern Pakistan. Archives of Ophthalmology. 2010;**128**(1):107-113

[17] Hameed A et al. A novel locus for Leber congenital amaurosis (LCA4) with anterior keratoconus mapping to chromosome 17p13. Investigative Ophthalmology & Visual Science. 2000;**41**(3):629-633

[18] Elder MJ. Leber congenital amaurosis and its association with keratoconus and keratoglobus. Journal of Pediatric Ophthalmology and Strabismus. 1994;**31**(1):38-40

[19] Stoiber J et al. Recurrent keratoconus in a patient with Leber

congenital amaurosis. Cornea. 2000;**19**(3):395-398

[20] Li SW et al. Clinical features of 233 cases of keratoconus. Zhonghua Yan Ke Za Zhi. 2005;**41**(7):610-613

[21] Wong V, Ho D. Ocular abnormalities in down syndrome: An analysis of 140 Chinese children. Pediatric Neurology. 1997;**16**(4):311-314

[22] Liza-Sharmini AT, Azlan ZN, Zilfalil BA. Ocular findings in Malaysian children with down syndrome. Singapore Medical Journal. 2006;**47**(1):14-19

[23] Kim JH et al. Characteristic ocular findings in Asian children with down syndrome. Eye. 2002;**16**(6):710-714

[24] Mas Tur V et al. A review of keratoconus: Diagnosis, pathophysiology, and genetics. Survey of Ophthalmology. 2017;**62**(6):770-783

[25] Wang YM et al. Comparison of corneal dynamic and tomographic analysis in normal, forme fruste keratoconic, and keratoconic eyes. Journal of Refractive Surgery. 2017;**33**(9):632-638

[26] Chan TCY et al. Comparison of corneal tomography and a new combined tomographic biomechanical index in subclinical keratoconus. Journal of Refractive Surgery. 2018;**34**(9):616-621

[27] Colin J et al. Correcting keratoconus with intracorneal rings. Journal of Cataract and Refractive Surgery. 2000;**26**(8):1117-1122

[28] Tu KL et al. Quantification of the surgically induced refractive effect of intrastromal corneal ring segments in keratoconus with standardized incision site and segment size. Journal of Cataract and Refractive Surgery. 2011;**37**(10):1865-1870

[29] Tan DT et al. Corneal transplantation. Lancet. 2012;**379**(9827):1749-1761

[30] Sarezky D et al. Trends in corneal transplantation in keratoconus. Cornea. 2017;**36**(2):131-137

[31] Sykakis E et al. Corneal collagen cross-linking for treating keratoconus. Cochrane Database of Systematic Reviews. 2015;**3**:CD010621

[32] Wittig-Silva C et al. A randomized, controlled trial of corneal collagen cross-linking in progressive keratoconus: Three-year results. Ophthalmology. 2014;**121**(4):812-821

[33] Wang YM et al. Shift in progression rate of keratoconus before and after epithelium-off accelerated corneal collagen crosslinking. Journal of Cataract and Refractive Surgery. 2017;**43**(7):929-936

[34] Fernandez Perez J, Valero Marcos A, Martinez Pena FJ. Early diagnosis of keratoconus: What difference is it making? The British Journal of Ophthalmology. 2014;**98**(11):1465-1466

[35] Ferdi AC et al. Keratoconus natural progression: A systematic review and meta-analysis of 11 529 eyes. Ophthalmology. 2019;**126**(7):935-945

[36] Khawaja AP et al. Genetic variants associated with corneal biomechanical properties and potentially conferring susceptibility to keratoconus in a genome-wide association study. JAMA Ophthalmology. 2019;**137**(9):1005-1012

[37] Krachmer JH, Feder RS, Belin MW. Keratoconus and related noninflammatory corneal thinning disorders. Survey of Ophthalmology. 1984;**28**(4):293-322

[38] Matthaei M et al. Changing indications in penetrating keratoplasty:

A systematic review of 34 years of global reporting. Transplantation. 2017;**101**(6):1387-1399

[39] Hashemi H et al. The prevalence and risk factors for keratoconus: A systematic review and meta-analysis. Cornea. 6 Sep 2019. [Online ahead of print]

[40] Kok YO, Tan GF, Loon SC. Review: Keratoconus in Asia. Cornea. 2012;**31**(5):581-593

[41] Reeves SW et al. Keratoconus in the medicare population. Cornea. 2009;**28**(1):40-42

[42] Nielsen K et al. Incidence and prevalence of keratoconus in Denmark. Acta Ophthalmologica Scandinavica. 2007;**85**(8):890-892

[43] Pearson AR et al. Does ethnic origin influence the incidence or severity of keratoconus? Eye. 2000;**14**:625-628

[44] Georgiou T et al. Influence of ethnic origin on the incidence of keratoconus and associated atopic disease in Asians and white patients. Eye. 2004;**18**(4):379-383

[45] Cozma I, Atherley C, James NJ. Influence of ethnic origin on the incidence of keratoconus and associated atopic disease in Asian and white patients. Eye. 2005;**19**(8):924-925; author reply 925-6

[46] Ziaei H et al. Epidemiology of keratoconus in an Iranian population. Cornea. 2012;**31**(9):1044-1047

[47] Hashemi H et al. High prevalence and familial aggregation of keratoconus in an Iranian rural population: A population-based study. Ophthalmic & Physiological Optics. 2018;**38**(4):447-455

[48] Assiri AA et al. Incidence and severity of keratoconus in

Asir province, Saudi Arabia. The British Journal of Ophthalmology. 2005;**89**(11):1403-1406

[49] Saini JS et al. Keratoconus in Asian eyes at a tertiary eye care facility. Clinical & Experimental Optometry. 2004;**87**(2):97-101

[50] Shetty R et al. Current review and a simplified "five-point management algorithm" for keratoconus. Indian Journal of Ophthalmology. 2015;**63**(1):46-53

[51] Jonas JB et al. Prevalence and associations of keratoconus in rural Maharashtra in Central India: The Central India eye and medical study. American Journal of Ophthalmology. 2009;**148**(5):760-765

[52] Ota R, Fujiki K, Nakayasu K. Estimation of patient visit rate and incidence of keratoconus in the 23 wards of Tokyo. Nippon Ganka Gakkai Zasshi. 2002;**106**(6):365-372

[53] Xu L et al. Prevalence and associations of steep cornea/keratoconus in greater Beijing. The Beijing eye study. PLoS One. 2012;**7**(7):e39313

[54] Pan CW et al. Ethnic variation in central corneal refractive power and steep cornea in Asians. Ophthalmic Epidemiology. 2014;**21**(2):99-105

[55] Vazirani J, Basu S. Keratoconus: Current perspectives. Clinical Ophthalmology. 2013;**7**:2019-2030

[56] Ertan A, Muftuoglu O. Keratoconus clinical findings according to different age and gender groups. Cornea. 2008;**27**(10):1109-1113

[57] Fink BA et al. Differences in keratoconus as a function of gender. American Journal of Ophthalmology. 2005;**140**(3):459-468

[58] Adachi W et al. The association of HLA with young-onset keratoconus in Japan. American Journal of Ophthalmology. 2002;**133**(4):557-559

[59] Owens H, Gamble G. A profile of keratoconus in New Zealand. Cornea. 2003;**22**(2):122-125

[60] Etzine S. Conical cornea in identical twins. South African Medical Journal. 1954;**28**(8):154-155

[61] Zadnik K, Mannis MJ, Johnson CA. An analysis of contrast sensitivity in identical twins with keratoconus. Cornea. 1984;**3**(2):99-103

[62] Bechara SJ, Waring GO 3rd, Insler MS. Keratoconus in two pairs of identical twins. Cornea. 1996;**15**(1):90-93

[63] McMahon TT et al. Discordance for keratoconus in two pairs of monozygotic twins. Cornea. 1999;**18**(4):444-451

[64] Tuft SJ et al. Keratoconus in 18 pairs of twins. Acta Ophthalmologica. 2012;**90**(6):e482-e486

[65] Zadnik K et al. Baseline findings in the collaborative longitudinal evaluation of keratoconus (CLEK) study. Investigative Ophthalmology & Visual Science. 1998;**39**(13):2537-2546

[66] Wagner H, Barr JT, Zadnik K. Collaborative longitudinal evaluation of keratoconus (CLEK) study: Methods and findings to date. Contact Lens & Anterior Eye. 2007;**30**(4):223-232

[67] Weed KH et al. The Dundee university Scottish keratoconus study: Demographics, corneal signs, associated diseases, and eye rubbing. Eye. 2008;**22**(4):534-541

[68] Sharma R et al. Clinical profile and risk factors for keratoplasty and development of hydrops in north Indian patients with keratoconus. Cornea. 2009;**28**(4):367-370

[69] Hashemi H et al. Corneal collagen cross-linking with riboflavin and ultraviolet a irradiation for keratoconus: Long-term results. Ophthalmology. 2013;**120**(8):1515-1520

[70] Valgaeren H, Koppen C, Van Camp G. A new perspective on the genetics of keratoconus: Why have we not been more successful? Ophthalmic Genetics. 2018;**39**(2):158-174

[71] Li X et al. Two-stage genome-wide linkage scan in keratoconus sib pair families. Investigative Ophthalmology & Visual Science. 2006;**47**(9):3791-3795

[72] Bisceglia L et al. Linkage analysis in keratoconus: Replication of locus 5q21.2 and identification of other suggestive loci. Investigative Ophthalmology & Visual Science. 2009;**50**(3):1081-1086

[73] Hutchings H et al. Identification of a new locus for isolated familial keratoconus at 2p24. Journal of Medical Genetics. 2005;**42**(1):88-94

[74] Brancati F et al. A locus for autosomal dominant keratoconus maps to human chromosome 3p14-q13. Journal of Medical Genetics. 2004;**41**(3):188-192

[75] Tang YG et al. Genomewide linkage scan in a multigeneration Caucasian pedigree identifies a novel locus for keratoconus on chromosome 5q14.3-q21.1. Genetics in Medicine. 2005;**7**(6):397-405

[76] Gajecka M et al. Localization of a gene for keratoconus to a 5.6-Mb interval on 13q32. Investigative Ophthalmology & Visual Science. 2009;**50**(4):1531-1539

[77] Tyynismaa H et al. A locus for autosomal dominant keratoconus:

Linkage to 16q22.3-q23.1 in finnish families. Investigative Ophthalmology & Visual Science. 2002;**43**(10):3160-3164

[78] Fullerton J et al. Identity-by-descent approach to gene localisation in eight individuals affected by keratoconus from north-West Tasmania, Australia. Human Genetics. 2002;**110**(5):462-470

[79] Lu Y et al. Genome-wide association analyses identify multiple loci associated with central corneal thickness and keratoconus. Nature Genetics. 2013;**45**(2):155-163

[80] Vithana EN et al. Collagen-related genes influence the glaucoma risk factor, central corneal thickness. Human Molecular Genetics. 2011;**20**(4):649-658

[81] Hoehn R et al. Population-based meta-analysis in Caucasians confirms association with COL5A1 and ZNF469 but not COL8A2 with central corneal thickness. Human Genetics. 2012;**131**(11):1783-1793

[82] Burdon KP et al. Association of polymorphisms in the hepatocyte growth factor gene promoter with keratoconus. Investigative Ophthalmology & Visual Science. 2011;**52**(11):8514-8519

[83] Dudakova L et al. Validation of rs2956540:G>C and rs3735520:G>A association with keratoconus in a population of European descent. European Journal of Human Genetics. 2015;**23**(11):1581-1583

[84] Sahebjada S et al. Association of the hepatocyte growth factor gene with keratoconus in an Australian population. PLoS One. 2014;**9**(1):e84067

[85] Bykhovskaya Y et al. Variation in the lysyl oxidase (LOX) gene is associated with keratoconus in family-based and case-control studies. Investigative

Ophthalmology & Visual Science. 2012;**53**(7):4152-4157

[86] Iglesias AI et al. Cross-ancestry genome-wide association analysis of corneal thickness strengthens link between complex and Mendelian eye diseases. Nature Communications. 2018;**9**(1):1864

[87] Han S et al. Association of variants in FRAP1 and PDGFRA with corneal curvature in Asian populations from Singapore. Human Molecular Genetics. 2011;**20**(18):3693-3698

[88] Chen P et al. CMPK1 and RBP3 are associated with corneal curvature in Asian populations. Human Molecular Genetics. 2014;**23**(22):6129-6136

[89] Guggenheim JA et al. A genome-wide association study for corneal curvature identifies the platelet-derived growth factor receptor alpha gene as a quantitative trait locus for eye size in white Europeans. Molecular Vision. 2013;**19**:243-253

[90] Mishra A et al. Genetic variants near PDGFRA are associated with corneal curvature in Australians. Investigative Ophthalmology & Visual Science. 2012;**53**(11):7131-7136

[91] Miyake M et al. Identification of myopia-associated WNT7B polymorphisms provides insights into the mechanism underlying the development of myopia. Nature Communications. 2015;**6**:6689

[92] Gao X et al. Genome-wide association study identifies WNT7B as a novel locus for central corneal thickness in Latinos. Human Molecular Genetics. 2016;**25**(22):5035-5045

[93] Cuellar-Partida G et al. WNT10A exonic variant increases the risk of keratoconus by decreasing corneal thickness. Human Molecular Genetics. 2015;**24**(17):5060-5068

[94] Li X et al. A genome-wide association study identifies a potential novel gene locus for keratoconus, one of the commonest causes for corneal transplantation in developed countries. Human Molecular Genetics. 2012;**21**(2):421-429

[95] Rong SS et al. Genetic associations for keratoconus: A systematic review and meta-analysis. Scientific Reports. 2017;7(1):4620

[96] Vitart V et al. New loci associated with central cornea thickness include COL5A1, AKAP13 and AVGR8. Human Molecular Genetics. 2010;**19**(21):4304-4311

[97] Lu Y et al. Common genetic variants near the brittle cornea syndrome locus ZNF469 influence the blinding disease risk factor central corneal thickness. PLoS Genetics. 2010;**6**(5):e1000947

[98] Saravani R et al. Evaluation of possible relationship between COL4A4 gene polymorphisms and risk of keratoconus. Cornea. 2015;**34**(3):318-322

[99] Kokolakis NS et al. Polymorphism analysis of COL4A3 and COL4A4 genes in Greek patients with keratoconus. Ophthalmic Genetics. 2014;**35**(4):226-228

[100] De Bonis P et al. Mutational screening of VSX1, SPARC, SOD1, LOX, and TIMP3 in keratoconus. Molecular Vision. 2011;**17**:2482-2494

[101] Heon E et al. VSX1: A gene for posterior polymorphous dystrophy and keratoconus. Human Molecular Genetics. 2002;**11**(9):1029-1036

[102] Li X et al. Genetic association of COL5A1 variants in keratoconus patients suggests a complex connection between corneal thinning and keratoconus. Investigative Ophthalmology & Visual Science. 2013;**54**(4):2696-2704

[103] Vincent AL et al. Mutations in the zinc finger protein gene, ZNF469, contribute to the pathogenesis of keratoconus. Investigative Ophthalmology & Visual Science. 2014;**55**(9):5629-5635

[104] Kim SH et al. Association of -31T>C and -511 C>T polymorphisms in the interleukin 1 beta (IL1B) promoter in Korean keratoconus patients. Molecular Vision. 2008;**14**:2109-2116

[105] Mikami T et al. Interleukin 1 beta promoter polymorphism is associated with keratoconus in a Japanese population. Molecular Vision. 2013;**19**:845-851

[106] Hasanian-Langroudi F et al. Association of Lysyl oxidase (LOX) polymorphisms with the risk of keratoconus in an Iranian population. Ophthalmic Genetics. 2015;**36**(4):309-314

[107] Palamar M et al. Relationship between IL1beta-511C>T and ILRN VNTR polymorphisms and keratoconus. Cornea. 2014;**33**(2):145-147

[108] Bisceglia L et al. VSX1 mutational analysis in a series of Italian patients affected by keratoconus: Detection of a novel mutation. Investigative Ophthalmology & Visual Science. 2005;**46**(1):39-45

[109] Shetty R et al. Two novel missense substitutions in the VSX1 gene: Clinical and genetic analysis of families with keratoconus from India. BMC Medical Genetics. 2015;**16**:33

[110] Wilson SE, Kim WJ. Keratocyte apoptosis: Implications on corneal wound healing, tissue organization, and disease. Investigative Ophthalmology & Visual Science. 1998;**39**(2):220-226

[111] Kim WJ et al. Keratocyte apoptosis associated with keratoconus.

Experimental Eye Research. 1999;**69**(5):475-481

[112] Wang Y et al. Association of interleukin-1 gene single nucleotide polymorphisms with keratoconus in Chinese Han population. Current Eye Research. 2016;**41**(5):630-635

[113] Cornes BK et al. Identification of four novel variants that influence central corneal thickness in multi-ethnic Asian populations. Human Molecular Genetics. 2012;**21**(2):437-445

[114] Sahebjada S et al. Evaluating the association between keratoconus and the corneal thickness genes in an independent Australian population. Investigative Ophthalmology & Visual Science. 2013;**54**(13):8224-8228

[115] Hao XD et al. Evaluating the association between keratoconus and reported genetic loci in a Han Chinese population. Ophthalmic Genetics. 2015;**36**(2):132-136

[116] Abu-Amero KK et al. Case-control association between CCT-associated variants and keratoconus in a Saudi Arabian population. Journal of Negative Results in Biomedicine. 2015;**14**:10

[117] Wang YM et al. Analysis of multiple genetic loci reveals MPDZ-NF1B rs1324183 as a putative genetic marker for keratoconus. The British Journal of Ophthalmology. 2018;**102**(12):1736-1741

[118] Stabuc-Silih M et al. Polymorphisms in COL4A3 and COL4A4 genes associated with keratoconus. Molecular Vision. 2009;**15**:2848-2860

[119] Sargazi S et al. Association of KIF26B and COL4A4 gene polymorphisms with the risk of keratoconus in a sample of Iranian population. International Ophthalmology. 2019;**39**(11):2621-2628

[120] Wang Y et al. Common single nucleotide polymorphisms and keratoconus in the Han Chinese population. Ophthalmic Genetics. 2013;**34**(3):160-166

[121] Loukovitis E et al. The proteins of keratoconus: A literature review exploring their contribution to the pathophysiology of the disease. Advances in Therapy. 2019;**36**(9):2205-2222

[122] Sykakis E et al. An in depth analysis of histopathological characteristics found in keratoconus. Pathology. 2012;**44**(3):234-239

[123] Meek KM et al. Changes in collagen orientation and distribution in keratoconus corneas. Investigative Ophthalmology & Visual Science. 2005;**46**(6):1948-1956

[124] Tuori AJ et al. The immunohistochemical composition of corneal basement membrane in keratoconus. Current Eye Research. 1997;**16**(8):792-801

[125] Joseph R, Srivastava OP, Pfister RR. Differential epithelial and stromal protein profiles in keratoconus and normal human corneas. Experimental Eye Research. 2011;**92**(4):282-298

[126] Maatta M et al. Differential expression of collagen types XVIII/endostatin and XV in normal, keratoconus, and scarred human corneas. Cornea. 2006;**25**(3):341-349

[127] Ghosh A et al. Proteomic and gene expression patterns of keratoconus. Indian Journal of Ophthalmology. 2013;**61**(8):389-391

[128] di Martino E, Ali M, Inglehearn CF. Matrix metalloproteinases in keratoconus - too much of a good thing? Experimental Eye Research. 2019;**182**:137-143

[129] Panahi Y et al. An analytical enrichment-based review of structural genetic studies on keratoconus. Journal of Cellular Biochemistry. 2019;**120**(4):4748-4756

[130] Pannebaker C, Chandler HL, Nichols JJ. Tear proteomics in keratoconus. Molecular Vision. 2010;**16**:1949-1957

[131] Balasubramanian SA et al. Proteases, proteolysis and inflammatory molecules in the tears of people with keratoconus. Acta Ophthalmologica. 2012;**90**(4):e303-e309

[132] Shetty R et al. Elevated expression of matrix metalloproteinase-9 and inflammatory cytokines in keratoconus patients is inhibited by cyclosporine a. Investigative Ophthalmology & Visual Science. 2015;**56**(2):738-750

[133] Lema I, Duran JA. Inflammatory molecules in the tears of patients with keratoconus. Ophthalmology. 2005;**112**(4):654-659

[134] Lema I et al. Subclinical keratoconus and inflammatory molecules from tears. The British Journal of Ophthalmology. 2009;**93**(6):820-824

[135] Sambursky R et al. Sensitivity and specificity of a point-of-care matrix metalloproteinase 9 immunoassay for diagnosing inflammation related to dry eye. JAMA Ophthalmology. 2013;**131**(1):24-28

[136] Wang YM et al. Analysis of multiple genetic loci reveals MPDZ-NF1B rs1324183 as a putative genetic marker for keratoconus. The British Journal of Ophthalmology. 2018;**102**(12):1736-1741

[137] Edwards M, McGhee CN, Dean S. The genetics of keratoconus. Clinical & Experimental Ophthalmology. 2001;**29**(6):345-351

[138] Hao XD et al. Decreased integrity, content, and increased transcript level of mitochondrial DNA are associated with keratoconus. PLoS One. 2016;**11**(10):e0165580

[139] Karolak JA et al. Evidence against ZNF469 being causative for keratoconus in polish patients. Acta Ophthalmologica. 2016;**94**(3):289-294

[140] Arbab M et al. TNF-alpha genetic predisposition and higher expression of inflammatory pathway components in keratoconus. Investigative Ophthalmology & Visual Science. 2017;**58**(9):3481-3487

[141] Liskova P et al. Replication of SNP associations with keratoconus in a Czech cohort. PLoS One. 2017;**12**(2):e0172365

[142] Guan T et al. Analysis of the VSX1 gene in sporadic keratoconus patients from China. BMC Ophthalmology. 2017;**17**(1):173

[143] Hao XD et al. De novo mutations of TUBA3D are associated with keratoconus. Scientific Reports. 2017;**7**(1):13570

[144] da Silva DC et al. Analysis of VSX1 variations in Brazilian subjects with keratoconus. J. Ophthalmic Vis. Res. 2018;**13**(3):266-273

[145] Lucas SEM et al. Rare, potentially pathogenic variants in 21 keratoconus candidate genes are not enriched in cases in a large Australian cohort of European descent. PLoS One. 2018;**13**(6):e0199178

[146] Zhang J et al. Evaluating the association between calpastatin (CAST) gene and keratoconus in the Han Chinese population. Gene. 2018;**653**:10-13